'Aafke Scharloo is a tireless pioneer, campaigner and clinician… Together with her two colleagues, Martine Spijker and Simone Ebbers, both psychologists, they have produced a major new book for the 21st century.'

*– from the Foreword by Valerie Sinason, PhD, MACP, M Inst Psychoanal, FIPD, Consultant Psychoanalyst and President of the Institute for Psychotherapy and Disability*

# PSYCHOLOGICAL FIRST AID

FOR PEOPLE WITH

# INTELLECTUAL DISABILITIES

WHO HAVE EXPERIENCED

# SEXUAL ABUSE

*of related interest*

**Learning Difficulties and Sexual Vulnerability**
**A Social Approach**
*Andrea Hollomotz*
ISBN 978 1 84905 167 5
eISBN 978 0 85700 381 2

**Sexuality and Relationships in the Lives of People with Intellectual Disabilities**
**Standing in My Shoes**
*Edited by Rohhss Chapman, Sue Ledger and Louise Townson with Daniel Docherty*
ISBN 978 1 84905 250 4
eISBN 978 0 85700 530 4

**Caring for the Physical and Mental Health of People with Learning Disabilities**
*David Perry, Louise Hammond, Geoff Marston, Sherryl Gaskell and James Eva*
*Foreword by Dr Anthony Kearns*
ISBN 978 1 84905 131 6
eISBN 978 0 85700 225 9

**Working with Adult Abuse**
**A Training Manual for People Working With Vulnerable Adults**
*Jacki Pritchard*
ISBN 978 1 84310 509 1
eISBN 978 1 84642 637 7

**Working with the Trauma of Rape and Sexual Violence**
**A Guide for Professionals**
*Sue J. Daniels*
*Foreword by Ivan Tyrell*
ISBN 978 1 78592 111 7
eISBN 978 1 78450 375 8

# PSYCHOLOGICAL FIRST AID FOR PEOPLE WITH INTELLECTUAL DISABILITIES WHO HAVE EXPERIENCED SEXUAL ABUSE

## A Step-by-Step Programme

AAFKE SCHARLOO,
SIMONE EBBERS AND
MARTINE SPIJKER

FOREWORD BY VALERIE SINASON

Jessica Kingsley *Publishers*
London and Philadelphia

First published in Dutch by Bohn Stafleu van Loghum in 2013
This edition first published in 2017
by Jessica Kingsley Publishers
73 Collier Street
London N1 9BE, UK
and
400 Market Street, Suite 400
Philadelphia, PA 19106, USA

*www.jkp.com*



**Library of Congress Cataloging in Publication Data**
Names: Scharloo, Aafke, author. | Ebbers, Simone, author. | Spijker, Martine, author.
Title: SOS, psychological first aid for people with intellectual disabilities after sexual abuse : a step-by-step programme / Aafke Scharloo, Simone Ebbers and Martine Spijker.
Other titles: SOS-snelle opvang bij seksueel misbruik van mensen met een verstandelijke beperking. English | Psychological first aid for people with intellectual disabilities after sexual abuse
Description: London ; Philadelphia : Jessica Kingsley Publishers, 2017. | Translation of: SOS-snelle opvang bij seksueel misbruik van mensen met een verstandelijke beperking / Drs. A. Scharloo, Drs. S. Ebbers, Drs. M. Spijker. Houten : Bohn Stafleu van Loghum, 2014. | Includes bibliographical references.
Identifiers: LCCN 2016025739 | ISBN 9781785921476 (alk. paper)
Subjects: | MESH: Crisis Intervention--methods | Mentally Disabled Persons--psychology | Sex Offenses--psychology | Psychological Trauma--rehabilitation | Intellectual Disability--psychology
Classification: LCC RC480.6 | NLM WM 401 | DDC 616.89/025--dc23 LC record available at https://lccn.loc.gov/2016025739

**British Library Cataloguing in Publication Data**
A CIP catalogue record for this book is available from the British Library

ISBN 978 1 78592 147 6
eISBN 978 1 78450 416 8

Printed and bound in Great Britain

MIX
Paper from responsible sources
FSC® C013056

# CONTENTS

# FOREWORD

In 1990 an historic international conference was held in the Netherlands. It was the first conference on the treatment of mental illness and behavioural disorder in people with intellectual disabilities. Došen, Van Gennep and Zwanniken were among the pioneers speaking at that conference and they later edited a book on the proceedings.[1] It was extremely moving to be present at that conference and receive emotional and clinical validation for speaking about sexual abuse and intellectual disability.

The Netherlands has a proud history of human rights and access to treatment of those with an intellectual disability, and nearly a quarter of a century later, a further major historic advance, the 2014 Dutch edition was the first book in the Netherlands to provide adequate tools to provide emotional first aid after disclosures of sexual abuse. It was an honour to write the foreword for such a crucial, timely and lifesaving book, and this English version allows even more readers to access this important information.

Across the world we continue to find it painful to acknowledge the extent of sexual abuse in our society. In the UK, the government estimate is that one in four people experience abuse at some point in their lifetime. Bowlby's seminal work (1979) highlighted for us already long ago the way illegitimate knowledge – knowledge which we are not supposed to have – leads to cognitive distortions.[2] When respected attachment figures offer danger to children and vulnerable adults we can become paralysed with inaction despite our awareness of the damage being caused.

As Ferenczi commented:[3]

> In the early states of embryonic development a slight wound, the mere prick of a pen, can not only cause severe alterations in, but may completely prevent, the development of whole limbs of the

body. Just as, if you have only one candle in a room and you put your hand near the candle, half the room may become darkened, so if, near the beginning of life, you do only a little harm to a child, it may cast a shadow over its entire life.

Learning disabled children are not only vulnerable to abuse in the way all children are, they are sadly more vulnerable precisely because of their communication problems, frequent lack of secure attachment, the societal unwillingness to consider that the most vulnerable citizens are also the most vulnerable to abuse and the way behaviour that communicates trauma is all too often misperceived as being due to the disability itself.

Physical and sexual abuse (which automatically includes emotional abuse) affects the body and mind of all children. Children with disabilities have added emotional vulnerability, which exacerbates the impact of abuse. Their frequent sense of being unwanted by society and their shame at their disability can make it harder for them to speak out.

Additionally, many have a fantasy that they are the products of a bad intercourse, which made them turn out wrong. This makes psychosexual development even harder.

Some can defend themselves from the trauma of their experience by creating a secondary handicap. This means that they exaggerate aspects of the real organic handicap to such an extent that the secondary handicap might even be more severe than the primary one.

The tragedy of this defence is that it depletes their emotional and cognitive resources. As part of such secondary defensive handicap many children and adults develop a falsely smiling face or manner under which they hide their pain and despair. The sense of loss and despair is thus hidden under the 'handicapped smile'.[4, 5]

Unfortunately, because so many carers and professionals cannot bear to deal with the emotional experience of learning disability the 'happy' expression is often responded to as if it was real. Alternatively, we see acts of major self-injury, inappropriate sexual behaviour and extreme sexual violence dismissed as being part of a disability rather than having meaning.

Against this, of course, it is important to remember the resilience of the constitutionally resilient child, especially the child whose disclosure is met with belief by their mother and others. It is also important, always, for us to remember the resilience of families and teams around a child or adult with a disability who have the emotional capacity to cope with trauma, especially if they are supported.

Aafke Scharloo is a tireless pioneer, campaigner and clinician, who has taken up these issues within the Netherlands and in Europe and America. Together with her two colleagues, Martine Spijker and Simone Ebbers, both psychologists, they have produced a major new book for the 21st century.

*Psychological First Aid* is indeed an apt title as it provides much-needed tools for an immediate response to a personal and public emergency. It involves carers and parents and is targeted to be helpful at all levels of disability.

*Valerie Sinason, PhD, MACP, M Inst Psychoanal, FIPD*

*Valerie Sinason is a Consultant Psychoanalyst and President of the Institute for Psychotherapy and Disability.*

# ACKNOWLEDGEMENTS

Writing this book has been a lengthy and inspiring process. We have worked on the text, together and individually, during many evenings and weekends. The process has been a great opportunity to deepen our knowledge of the literature on the subject and to sharpen our thought processes. Many discussions have been held and the result is finally here in print. We have sought theoretical inspiration from three main persepctives while writing this book.

First, we visited a worldwide conference about sexual abuse and maltreatment in San Diego a few years ago and came into contact with the American theory of 'Psychological First Aid'. The emphasis of this theory lies on the importance of good initial support for the coping process after shocking incidents. We soon realised that support such as this could be of great importance in preventing traumas for people with an intellectual disability who have experienced sexual abuse. And so the idea for this book was born.

In order to find a suitable form for the contents of the book, we then researched standard first support programmes and methods for coping with trauma in general terms. We have been inspired by the work of Mittendorf, Kleber, Boon, Steel, Van der hart, Brière and Perry. And finally, to refine our research for the target group of people with an intellectual disability, we consulted the work of Došen and of our English colleagues, including Sinason, Cottis and Hollins, who have been pioneers for so many years in the field of support and therapy for people with an intellectual disability who have been sexually abused. In addition, many other publications have been of direct and indirect value (see the references). Our aim was to connect the information from the various sources, and this book is the end result.

In writing this book we have received help and support from various people and organisations. We would like to take the opportunity of thanking them here. In the first place, our thanks go out to all the clients, care teams and colleagues who have shared their experiences with us and provided us with feedback on the support which they received from us. We have learnt so much from them and it is partly due to them that this book is now here. We would also like to thank the parents and relatives who have provided us with feedback. A special word of thanks to Jannes and Eelkje de Jong, who, as experienced parents, not only shared their experiences with us but also gave us feedback on the chapter about parents.

Many more people have helped along the way. We would like to thank everyone for their help, especially Kreel de Leeuw, our colleague and dedicated adviser. With her sharp insight, she has provided feedback on various chapters. Thanks to Reinout Lievegoed for the advice and for reading the part about trauma processing in people with an intellectual disability, and to Lilian van der Leeuw from Prima Assistentie who assisted us by day and by night in preparing the manuscript. We would have never have made the deadline without her help.

We are especially grateful to Ferdinand Bennink, who frequently made his beautiful house in Germany available for us so that we could work on this book in peaceful and pleasant surroundings.

Finally, a special word of thanks to our husbands (Noel, Jacco and Michiel) and children (Floor, Robin, Sam, Cas, Nikai and Jade). They have stood by us, given us courage and had to do without us at the most inconvenient times. Now we have time for them again!

# GENERAL INTRODUCTION

This handbook is the result of many years work with people with an intellectual disability who have experienced sexual abuse and their families. The methods provided have evolved from our experience of working with this group of people and also from literary study of the growing number of publications in the field of support after trauma and coping with trauma, which have proved very useful and relevant in our work. In addition, we have also learnt a great deal from the clients themselves, their parents and relatives and the various teams we have worked with. They have all overcome difficulties again and again and, despite everything, have shown much trust and have been able to share their experiences with us. We owe these people our greatest respect. With this handbook we hope to be able to share the lessons they have taught us so that others too can benefit from them.

Working with people with an intellectual disability who have been made victim of sexual abuse and maltreatment is emotionally challenging and difficult for all those involved. Whereas before the abuse was disclosed, everyone was able to act on the basis of the care/support/treatment/development plan, after the disclosure of abuse there is suddenly an overwhelming sense of powerlessness and uncertainty, which can have a numbing effect. Nothing is quite as it was before...

Sexual abuse occurs frequently in people with an intellectual disability compared with others in our society. Due to the high prevalence of abuse, you may expect care providers and other organisations who work with people with an intellectual disability to be well prepared for psychological first aid support and care for people who have experienced such incidents. However, this is not always the case. People are often unsure of how to act and, in practice, it appears that structured support and guidance for people with an intellectual disability (and their parents and relatives) after overwhelming incidents of this sort are scarce.

Fortunately, there is often attention given to the issues surrounding sexual abuse. Many institutions apply a reporting code and a quality action protocol for incidents of sexual abuse. Nevertheless, most professionals and managers feel insuffiently comfortable with issues concerning sexual abuse and the support of people after such an overwhelming incident, and are not well prepared to direct this process in the right way. Organisational issues also play a role (whose task is it, how much time is available?) and there seems to be tension between support for the client and good healthcare professionalism on the one hand, and the investigation and/or legal course of action on the other hand. Support in the coping process is sometimes delayed because of the investigation. The advice is often given in the case of criminal investigations to talk as little as possible with the client about what has happened.

It is evident that not talking about what has happened is not beneficial for the coping process, certainly if the police investigation takes a long time. In literature on the subject of coping with shocking events, emphasis is given to the importance of providing help as soon as possible due to the fact that people struggle with important questions and strong, overwhelming emotions in the initial period. In practice, the client finds themselves in limbo when they have to wait for the police process, waiting lists, and when there are limited opportunities for therapy. Clients can seem to be in a vacuum, where no one knows quite what to do. At the very moment that the needs are greatest, clients experience the most confusion, loneliness and the feeling of having to deal with things on their own. This handbook has been designed to change this situation. The book provides professionals with various guidelines by which to provide professional and structured help for clients during this difficult period.

The book begins with a general description of the SOS programme. This includes the contents of the programme and a description of the target group. The importance of starting with the programme straightaway is explained from the perspective of the clients themselves, their parents and relatives and also for the team of professional caregivers. An overview is also given of the main points of the programme. A number of general chapters follow, in which the issues surrounding sexual abuse of people with an intellectual disability are discussed.

- Chapter 2 describes the prevalence, the integrated ecological theory and the implications of sexual abuse for people with an intellectual disability.
- In Chapter 3, legal boundaries and other relevant issues are addressed. Attention is paid to minimum fact interviews, the course of action regarding the police, and dealing with the media.
- Chapter 4 describes trauma and the process of coping with trauma. Age-specific stress reactions and the way in which people with an intellectual disability cope with trauma are addressed here.
- Chapter 5 focuses on support for people with an intellectual disability who have been sexually abused. Preparation and points of attention are discussed, alongside the structure and contents of the client sessions and the function of the help book.
- Chapter 6 describes the support of people with a mild to moderate intellectual disability. Specific issues related to developmental stages are addressed for both groups, and exercises are given for the support of these groups of people after sexual abuse.
- Chapter 7 focuses on people with a severe intellectual disability and sexual abuse. Here it is emphasised that in the support of these clients, the recovery of safety and relationships is a central theme as a way to calm the stress response system. The support sessions are described and suggestions for practical exercises are given.
- Chapter 8 focuses on the support of parents and relatives of clients who have been sexually abused. There is attention for the special connection which people with an intellectual disability have with their parents and the implications of these dynamics for the coping process after abuse, for both the parents and the client.

- Chapter 9 describes the support for the team of professional caregivers and the processes that play a role here. A description is given of the best way to support the client in their daily life and the ways in which the caregivers can support the parents. There is also attention for team processes such as splitting, transference and countertransference. Finally, signalling secondary traumatising, as a consequence of working with people who have experienced serious incidents, is described, making it possible to react in an appropriate manner at any stage.
- Chapter 10 contains methods and exercises to help parents, relatives and the team of caregivers during the SOS programme.

This book provides diverse literary references. These are intended as further reading material for the professional.

The downloadable materials in Chapters 6, 7 and 10 can be accessed online at www.jkp.com/voucher using the code SCHARLOOPSYCHAID.

Working in the field of psychological first aid support for people with an intellectual disability who have been sexually abused, and their systems, can be heavy and exhausting work. It can, however, also be extremely satisfying. It is beautiful to see how people with a relatively simple support programme such as this are able to pick up the pieces and get back to daily life again, together with others. We hope that the SOS programme – alongside the practical tools provided – can also give other colleagues in the field the same experience.

## Chapter 1

# THE SOS HANDBOOK

## PSYCHOLOGICAL FIRST AID AFTER SEXUAL ABUSE

### Introduction

Sexual abuse of children, young people and adults with an intellectual disability can present professional caregivers and others surrounding the victim with feelings of confusion and powerlessness. A research report into the prevalence of sexual abuse in an institution for people with an intellectual disability once bore the title 'impossibly true',[1] as a reference to a statement made by a respondent who aptly described the feelings arising from the issue. People around the victim sway back and forth between the will to deny and the will to rush to help. Dealing with sexual abuse, however, requires thoughtful action, which is not a simple task when people find themselves in a state of confusion.[2]

Fortunately, care organisations possess protocols and guidelines in which step-by-step actions are described. Codes for reporting and protocols concerning (suspected) sexual abuse provide many practical guidelines about how to act immediately after (suspicion of) sexual abuse has come to light.

Alongside practical action there is also a great need for adequate psychological support in the following period. Until now this been limited, although countless scientific research reports from the past 20 years show that such support is essential for the coping process of those involved.[3] With regard to issues around sexual abuse, many professionals and managers do not feel sufficiently capable of effectively implementing support for those involved after such experiences. If a police statement takes place, there seems to be tension between the support of the client and good professional care on the one hand, and the police investigation and/or the legal process on the other hand. This handbook provides concrete measures for making first aid support possible for clients and their systems (parents, relatives and the care team).

## 1.1 Target group of the SOS handbook

The SOS handbook has been developed for victims (both children and adults) of sexual abuse who have an intellectual disability. In the support of these victims it is important to make a distinction between clients who have experienced sexual abuse once and clients who have repeatedly been sexually abused over a longer period of time.

In the first case, the client is overwhelmed by the incident. A single incident of sexual abuse takes place so unexpectedly that the client cannot use defence mechanisms. A sense of powerlessness and disruption is experienced. In this case, the client usually recovers from the most serious symptoms within half a year, with the help of a safe and supporting environment.

In cases of long-term sexual abuse, multiple incidents of sexual abuse, and in situations involving violence or threats of violence, the client will often have developed defence reactions. The client will have needed these reactions in order to tackle the abusive situation and to protect themselves against painful experiences. This can include avoidance reactions, identity problems, relationship problems and difficulty with regulating emotions (lack of feeling, strong emotions and/or depression).[4] These reactions are often deeply embedded in the behavioural pattern and are not easy to change. In most cases of sexual abuse involving people with an intellectual disability, the abuse has been taking place for a longer period of time. It is also known that people with an intellectual disability stand a higher chance than others of becoming more frequent victims of sexual abuse.[5] This means that new situations of abuse will often cause memories of earlier abuse to arise and even more overwhelming symptoms to occur. Chapter 2 addresses the prevalence and causes of sexual abuse concerning people with an intellectual disability.

The SOS handbook can be used in situations of single or multiple abuse. It is possible that using this book will be sufficient for the victim to be able to resume daily life again. This will most surely not be the case for the second category of clients. Long-term therapy aimed at treating chronic trauma is generally indicated in such cases.

The SOS handbook has been written for the support of the client with an intellectual disability. The programme makes a distinction between clients with a severe intellectual disability (IQ 0–35), clients with a moderate intellectual disability (IQ 35–50) and those with a mild intellectual disability (IQ 50–70 or 70–85).

The programme can be used for clients of all ages; the help book provides exercises which are adapted for the various levels of cognitive functioning and range of ages. A selection should be made from the various exercises, depending on the situation of the specific client. It goes without saying that not only the cognitive level of functioning should be taken into account when choosing the exercises.

The SOS handbook has been developed for the support of people with an intellectual disability who have been sexually abused. The method is – with a few small adaptations – also suitable to use for people with an intellectual disability who have experienced other forms of abuse, such as physical or emotional maltreatment.

## 1.2 The importance of the system

The SOS handbook is not only aimed at supporting the client with an intellectual disability: the programme also includes sessions with the parents/guardians and professional caregivers as well as with the client themselves. Significant others in the life of a person with an intellectual disability are referred to in the book by the collective term 'system'.

Almost everybody who has been confronted by sexual abuse in their surrounding environment is affected by it. This is definitely true for parents/guardians. A process of support and guidance is needed, aimed at the consequences for them – in their role as parent and in the caring for/upbringing of their child. Incidents of abuse also affect the professional caregivers involved to such an extent that support in coping with the situation is required. In addition, they often need support for a longer period of time in order to be able to care for the client adequately and not become caught up in their own transfer responses, which are unavoidable in working with victims of sexual abuse. The personal process of the parents/carers and professional caregivers involved also plays a crucial role in the recovery process of the client. Research shows that coping with sexual abuse for a person with an intellectual disability is strongly connected to the way in which significant others cope with the abuse.[6] This is logical when considering the relational and environmental dependence in which people with an intellectual disability function. Many people with an intellectual disability have a close emotional connection to their family, often into old age, as this is the constant factor in their lives.

Also in the case of adults of all ages with an intellectual disability, the parents/guardians and professional caregivers play a crucial role in coping with the situation. The lower the victim's level of functioning, the more the emphasis lies on the 'coping interventions' of the surrounding system.

## 1.3 Task of the professional

The SOS handbook has been written for the professional who works in the care and support of people with an intellectual disability. We have chosen to assign this task to the professional as, due to their training, this group is sufficiently qualified to provide this type of help. Additionally, their position makes them sufficiently involved with the client, but at enough of a distance so as not to be too much a part of the system. This professional distance is necessary in order to be able to adequately deal with the emotions of those involved.

However, if there is not an adequate professional distance, then the SOS programme should not be performed by this person but instead by a professional colleague. In order to clearly apply this programme, the attitude of the practitioner is critically important. A direct and inviting attitude is needed, in which the process is initiated in a structured manner and a feeling of safety for people who are upset (by what they have experienced) is created. It is also important that the practitioner is aware of the fact that they will be functioning as a role model for those involved. The subject of sexual abuse is often burdened with shame and silence. Demonstrating an active approach, which does not avoid explicit discussion of the issues, will help those involved to express their experiences and emotions. It is also important to show kindness and capability, and to state that nothing is too crazy to talk about and that absolutely everything can be said. It helps clients to know that their professional often talks to people who have been sexually abused and they are not the only one in this situation! It is the task of the practitioner to ensure an atmosphere which is not too strongly emotionally charged. For this purpose it helps to use (suitable) humour.

The fact that this programme has been written for professionals does not mean that we assume that they will conduct the programme alone. We emphasise the fact that dealing with situations of sexual abuse requires a multidisciplinary approach. When this includes support for the professional caregivers involved, the tasks and close involvement of the responsible manager is certainly also required!

---

It is essential that the organisation ensures that the professional is facilitated in conducting the programme. It is recommended to include the SOS programme in the organisation's vision and policy on sexual abuse.

---

## 1.4 Aims of the SOS handbook

The SOS handbook has been developed as a first aid programme in the support of (or involvement with) people with an intellectual disability who have been made victims of sexual abuse. The SOS programme is emphatically *not* meant to replace later treatment or therapy. It is a guideline for conduct, after a report has been made according to the reporting code and/or protocol in (suspected) sexual abuse.

The SOS programme is immediately implemented after the disclosure or discovery of a situation (or suspicion) of sexual abuse. Research shows that fast and active intervention initiated by third parties proves most effective in guiding and benefiting the coping process.[7] Using the SOS handbook can prevent or break through the isolation of the victim or system. It provides a safe situation for the client in which they can 'talk' about what has happened and where all doubts and concerns can be expressed. In using this programme, it is possible to help those involved to tolerate and order primary stress reactions as a consequence of sexual abuse. The natural coping process is supported and this prevents the process stagnating, with all of the consequences this brings. At the same time it is also possible to consider the type, intensity and progress of the stress reactions. Possible problems can be recognised at an early stage, making adequate responses possible.

The SOS handbook can be used after a disclosure and/or discovery of a situation of (suspected) sexual abuse. Those involved sometimes think that sexual abuse should first be proved before taking action. The fact that it may not yet have been proved does not actually mean that professional caregivers cannot do their work. The perceptual experience of suspected victims can be supported without evidence or a judicial ruling.[8]

## 1.5 Structure of the SOS handbook

Prior to the practical layout of the sessions, three chapters of background information are provided which the professional must be aware of before conducting the programme.

- Chapter 2 describes the prevalence, definition and implication of sexual abuse in people with an intellectual disability.
- Chapter 3 contains information about reporting codes, protocols, law and regulations, minimum fact interviews, statements (or reports) to the police, medical examinations and dealing with the media.
- Chapter 4 provides background information about types of trauma, the neurobiological aspects of trauma, trauma reactions, secondary traumatising, and coping with trauma. Special attention is paid to trauma and coping with trauma in people with an intellectual disability.

The SOS programme focuses on the client, the parents/carers or other significant people and also the professional caregivers involved. The starting point is that the client's next of kin, according to the protocol in sexual abuse, have been informed about the sexual abuse or the suspicion of such. The professional organises four sessions for each of the three different target groups (client, parents/carers and professional caregivers). The conversations with the client take approximately 45 minutes, depending on the capacity and concentration ability of the client.

For the sessions with the parents and the team, approximately 90 minutes are required per session.

The first contact takes place as soon as possible, preferably within a week after the disclosure/discovery (and after the minimum fact interview). The second session follows about a week later. The first two sessions with those involved take place independently: a session with the client, a session with the parents/carers and a session with the professional caregivers involved. The third session is a joint session in which the client, their system and the professional caregivers involved share their experiences and (learn to) communicate with each other about what has happened. This joint session is planned approximately a month after the start of the programme. After eight weeks there is a follow-up session for each group independently.

A detailed plan for each session is given in the SOS handbook. Points of attention and exercises that can help with communication and coping with the needs of the victim are described. The contents are based on insights from literature regarding support after trauma, sexual abuse and trauma treatment for people with and without an intellectual disability, added to by insights which have arisen from practical experience.

The order and content of the subjects of the sessions have been chosen on the basis of literature and experience. It is important that the professional realises that flexibility in implementing the SOS programme is possible and can even be necessary, depending on the situation. The programme is therefore not a protocol or compulsory 'straightjacket', but instead a guideline. The SOS handbook can be added to and adapted using personal creativity, according to the actual circumstances. The different developmental levels have been taken into account in the individual sessions with the client. Using flexibility and creativity is recommended in order to adapt the sessions to the situation and needs of the individual client.

## 1.6 The SOS help books

Alongside information about trauma and coping with trauma with regard to people with an intellectual disability, the SOS handbook includes practical advice for supporting those involved. Help books have been developed for each target group. The help book for the client provides exercises, adapted to the level of functioning, which enable the incidents (and the perception of them) to be 'discussed', understood and ordered. These exercises are categorised according to the trauma-related themes: safety, worries, hurt, fear, anger, relaxation and survival.[9] The exercises given differ for levels of cognitive functioning: mild, moderate and severely intellectually disabled. Exercises are given in the last chapter for the support of parents and the client's professional caregivers. For the professional caregivers there are exercises which focus on the personal coping process of the individual caregiver and also of the care team.

The help book pays attention to the personal coping process of the parent/professional caregiver, in addition to the importance of the role of the parent/professional caregiver in the coping process of the victim of sexual abuse.

Alongside the exercises, material is provided which can be used for psychoeducation on sexual abuse and coping with trauma. Practical information has also been included about making a police statement, studio hearing and dealing with the media. The help book has been designed so that the contents can be adapted for the individual client, those involved and the incident of abuse.

## 1.7 What to do in the case of serious problems after completion of the SOS programme

After completion of the SOS programme, a decrease in symptoms is usually observed. The incident itself is central at the start of the programme and those involved (the client and also parents/relatives and the professional care team) are often constantly consciously or subconsciously aware of it. Intrusions, nightmares and imposing memories often occur. The victim suffers avoidance behaviour or emotional numbness and there can be increased alertness and irritability. This lessens within time and these problems usually clearly lessen or largely disappear after about three months.

Victims of sexual abuse mainly suffer trauma type II (see Chapter 4); they usually need long-term intensive therapy. In the last session, just as in the other sessions, a check is preformed to assess the situation concerning these symptoms. Fast referral to therapeutic treatment is required if there is an increase of trauma-related symptoms in a person involved, or if the symptoms remain the same.

In order to be able to provide adequate therapy, a respected diagnostic course of action is sometimes required, which focuses on assessing the consequences of the trauma. In establishing the progress of the symptoms, it is important to not only consider the personal reports of the various people involved but also for people to be able to look objectively at their own symptoms. It is advisable to ask others involved how they view the situation. Experience teaches that clients are surprisingly good at perceiving how their parents/carers and professional caregivers are feeling. This means that clients also play an important role in assessing the well-being of those around them.

## 1.8 Care for yourself as implementer of the SOS handbook

Dealing with situations of sexual abuse and supporting those involved is a task which can have great impact. Meeting and empathising with people who have experienced shocking incidents also makes the professional caregiver vulnerable toward the effects of the incident. This can happen to everyone.

The professional, as implementer of the SOS programme, will at times feel powerless and angry, particularly when confronted by the intense stories of clients and their system and of colleagues. It is also possible that personal experiences from their own past will come to the surface. This can be painful and may emerge as a complete surprise.

It is important to be aware of the personal impact this work can have and to take possible stress symptoms seriously. It is difficult to conduct the SOS programme (and the required attitude aspects) if the person who is conducting the programme is overwhelmed by their own worries and exhaustion and as a result has less energy and strength. In order to prevent symptoms arising, peer-to-peer coaching, personal coaching and self-care are essential. Sharing experiences and seeking support from colleagues are of great importance in working with traumatised clients. It is also advisable to offer professionals coaching, with the emphasis on the emotional impact of working with traumatised people.

## SUMMARY

The SOS handbook focuses on professionals who work in the care and support of people with an intellectual disability. The SOS programme provides practical guidelines in order to make adequate first aid support possible for clients and their systems. This requires a multidisciplinary approach, close involvement of the manager and embedding in the organisation.

The SOS programme is designed to be used as a follow-up to a report of (suspected) sexual abuse according to a reporting code and/or protocol in sexual abuse, such as is implemented by many care providers for people with an intellectual disability. The SOS handbook is not a replacement for possible later treatment.

Adequate support of a victim of sexual abuse with an intellectual disability includes individual support for the client, but also for their system. The programme offers specific practical advice for clients of different cognitive levels, their parents/carers and professional caregivers. Help books are made for the support of each target group, containing practical exercises and useful information. The goal is to help people who have been involved in a situation of sexual abuse with the process of coping. They are supported in ordering, understanding and managing the situation and their own (stress) reactions.

Finally, it is important that attention is given to the support of the professional during the implementation of the SOS programme. Sharing experiences and seeking support from colleagues is extremely important when working with traumatised clients. Possible stress symptoms must be taken seriously; peer-to-peer coaching, personal coaching and self-care are essential as preventative measures.

Chapter 2

# SEXUAL ABUSE OF PEOPLE WITH AN INTELLECTUAL DISABILITY

## EXPLANATION AND DEFINITION

### Introduction

Various laws and regulations play a role in responding to incidents of sexual abuse in people with an intellectual disability. Professional caregivers often feel unsure of how to act, largely due to their limited knowledge in this field. In this chapter, attention is paid to the definition of sexual abuse, from both the psychological and the legal perspective. A short description is given of legal articles that are applicable in incidents of sexual abuse involving people with an intellectual disability. This does not only concern the type of sexual acts and the age of those involved, but also the victim's ability to give consent – an issue which plays a central role in legal cases concerning sexual abuse, as well as in other cases.

Additionally, this chapter describes the prevalence of sexual abuse in people with an intellectual disability. An analysis of the most influential models of explanation for the fact that people with an intellectual disability run a heightened risk of becoming a victim of sexual abuse is described in the integrated ecological theory of Sobsey. Sobsey emphasises that there is no causal relationship between having an intellectual disability and being a victim of sexual abuse. He states that people with intellectual disabilities are abused more often then others as a result of characteristics of the care system. These characteristics can be seen as risk factors strengthening each other.

The last part of the chapter addresses the specific implications and consequences of sexual abuse in people with an intellectual disability and their system.

## 2.1 The definition of sexual abuse

Sexual abuse is a broad concept. It can vary from being forced to endure sexual acts and perform them on others to being forced to perform them on oneself. Sexual abuse can also involve being made to watch the sexual acts of others or look at pornographic material which is not suitable for the age or developmental level of the victim.

There is a difference in power between the perpetrator and victim in every form of sexual abuse. This power difference can be due to the age, difference in developmental level, physical strength and difference in position of power as a result of a dependency relationship. A perpetrator can exert their influence in various ways. It often happens subtly, by paying the victim attention and giving presents or by isolating them and making them dependent. Sometimes, perpetrators may also use less subtle forms of force, such as threats of violence, emotional or psychological pressure or blackmail to force the victim to perform sexual acts and/or to keep them a secret.

Sexual contact between a person with an intellectual disability and a person without an intellectual disability is not by definition sexual abuse. We assume that people with an intellectual disability have the right to sexuality and their personal sexual experience and that they can make their own choices about this.[1] The precondition is that they are able to give consent concerning the sexual contact. The term 'consent' is important in understanding sexual violence in people with an intellectual disability. Definitions of sexual abuse in people with an intellectual disability are often based on not being able – or not wanting – to give consent for sexual contact.

Exploitation and safety are important concepts within the issue of consent.[2] McCarthy and Thompson have summarised the various attempts at making a definition by saying that sexual abuse happens 'where sexual acts are performed on or with someone who is unwilling or unable to consent to those acts', where 'any sexual contact which is unwanted and/or un-enjoyed by one partner and is for the sexual gratification of the other', and where 'that person's apparent willingness is unacceptably exploited'.[3]

## 2.2 Complex dynamics

Sexual abuse is a subject which gives rise to intense reactions. It is hard for us to believe that people whom we know and trust could do such things. Violence perpetrated by a person towards a usually weaker person is at odds with all of our values, norms and primitive defence mechanisms. Many people react in a defensive way to suspicions of abuse. In incidents of sexual abuse it is relatively easy to deny that it has happened as there is seldom actual evidence to be found. Due to the fact that sexual abuse (especially in people with an intellectual disability) usually comes to light much later on, there are generally no useable traces. In most cases there are no witnesses who have actually seen the sexual abuse.

### 2.2.1 The splitting phenomenon

A common defence mechanism, which especially starts working in cases of sexual abuse, is 'splitting'. Splitting occurs when an individual is not able to integrate something which is overwhelming or threatening. It not only occurs in individuals but is also often seen in teams, organisations and society concerning integrating intense events. In this more interactional definition, the term 'splitting' is used to convey the way in which a situation of sexual abuse can cause opposing and antagonising feelings and behaviour in a team or organisation. The splitting usually progresses along the lines of good-bad, sympathy-irritation, stating boundaries-emotional closeness, perpetrators-victims, believers and non-believers.[4]

In practice, splitting means that people choose a side; it works in a disruptive way. Camps form, which each concentrate on their own problem. In this way, the parties, in a subconscious and undeliberate way, are driven further apart. This complex dynamic means that the actions of those involved stem from emotions. This can lead to risky situations, in which disclosures and signs which victims give are not taken seriously or are interpreted wrongly. Suspected victims are sometimes not believed, suspected perpetrators are sometimes wrongly stigmatised or actual perpetrators are not recognised as being so.[5]

This unavoidably leads to inadequate action. The unity of parents and professional caregivers involved can be put under extreme pressure and can even lead to conflicts with one another, which has a destructive effect on the support of victim of the sexual abuse.

Using a protocol lessens the chance of splitting. We refer here to the reporting code, reporting obligation and the use of a protocol in (suspected) sexual abuse (see Section 3.1).

---

We emphasise the preventative effect of a safe social environment, in which communication is open and transparent and there is space for the different perceptions of the situation of those involved.

---

## 2.3 Sexual abuse and the law

In the Dutch Code of Criminal Procedure (Nederlandse Wetboek van Strafrecht) various articles have been included concerning sexual abuse.

Rape is described in article 246 as:

- Forcing someone by violence or another act to perpetrate or tolerate lewd actions.

Rape is defined in article 242 as:

- Forcing someone with violence or another act or threats of violence or another act to undergo actions which comprise of or partially comprise of sexually penetrating the body.

In article 244, sex with children under 12 years of age is forbidden. Article 245 forbids lewd actions with children under 16 years of age. In fact, this makes all sexual acts with children under 16 years of age illegal, and includes desired contact between two 15-year-olds. In practice, sexual contact between age group peers which takes place with mutual agreement is not prosecuted.

Since the abolition of the brothel ban in 2000, facilitating prostitution in the under-aged is no longer illegal. It is illegal to force prostitution on someone under 16 years of age (article 273f) and to use the prostitution services and facilities of a person younger than 16 years old.

It can be the case, also in the Netherlands, that children are used for pornographic material, often in combination with prostitution. In 2002, the laws for producing and possessing child pornographic material were tightened, making, distributing and possessing virtual child porn illegal (article 240b). Showing pornographic material to children is also illegal (article 240a).

Article 249 describes lewd behaviour concerning the abuse of authority and trust, in which conducting sexual acts within a power relationship and professional care relationship is illegal.

### 2.3.1 Legal status of people with an intellectual disability

All over the world there are laws to protect children and vulnerable adults against sexual abuse. However, in many countries the legal status of people with an intellectual disability who have been sexually abused is not strong at all. For people with intellectual disabilities, the bar has been set high to disclose what has happened to them. Legal systems seem to prefer victims who are verbal and open and are able to tell others what has happened. This leaves a lot of people with intellectual disabilities behind. This is a barrier to equal justice.

In addition, many people with intellectual disabilities have a limited ability to determine their own will, give consent and restrain from undesired contact. Because of the lack of protective laws in some countries, sexual abuse of people with intellectual disabilities is legally considered to be in mutual consent. The assumption is that people with an intellectual disability, when they have reached an adult age and no far-reaching protective measures have been made, are capable of giving informed consent and are therefore automatically considered to be legally able to restrain from undesired contact with any other adults.

In practice this means that not every form of sexual abuse of people with an intellectual disability can actually be classed as illegal. Think, for example, of situations in which perpetrators refer to the fact that they were not aware of the disability of the victim and therefore, when this cannot be proved otherwise, often get away with it because, legally speaking (even when the victim is not able to determine his or her own will), this would then be classed as sexual contact with mutual consent.

Although there is an apparent European obligation on this matter, not all European countries have legislation to protect vulnerable adult against these types of threat.

In England and Wales, a law has been in place since 2005 regarding the protection of vulnerable adults with an intellectual or psychiatric disbility: The Mental Capacity Act (see Box 2.1).[6]

### Box 2.1 Informed consent according to the Mental Capacity Act

In the Mental Capacity Act it is roughly stated that four aspects must be met if someone is to be defined as being able to give informed (sexual) consent.

1. The person must be able to make a distinction between important information and unimportant information regarding the decision to be made.
2. The person must be able to keep/remember (for a sufficient length of time) the information which is relevant in making the decision.
3. The person must be able to use and weigh up (oversee the consequences) the information as part of the process of decision making.
4. The person must be able to communicate the decision in whichever way possible.

## 2.3.2 Legal vs. clinical evidence

In contradiction to the legal definition of sexual abuse, which considers the objective facts, the subjective experience of the client forms the basis for implementing professional care. In professional care the experience of the client is always the starting point, even when the actual investigation has not (yet) taken place.[7]

In addition, it is important to make a definition between legally proved sexual abuse and clinically proved sexual abuse. Sexual abuse is only legally proved when it results in a prosecution within a criminal legal procedure. Sexual abuses can be considered clinically proved when two healthcare psychologists independently describe behavioural signals from clients as indicative of sexual abuse.

The term 'clinically proved' is mainly used so that people no longer talk about 'suspicions' in these cases, and so that clients and relatives can be supported more adequately in a manner which does justice to perception and experience. A term such as 'clinically proved' also legitimises taking safety measures, while a term such as 'suspicions' usually does not inspire people to actually take action and professional caregivers again and again get caught up in discussions and splitting phenomena, often at the expense of the interests of the client (see Sections 2.2.1 and 9.1.6).

## 2.4 Informed sexual consent

Informed sexual consent implies the level of understanding and ability to use the information and/or knowledge which is necessary to make a voluntary decision free from force. In the Dutch Medical Treatment Contracts Act it is stated that:

> A person can give informed consent when they are able to make a reasonable assessment of his or her relevant needs, in which attention must be paid to the context dependence of the term informed consent.[8]

Relevant here means: the subject about which the person is (un) able to give informed consent.[9] In the *Provisional Guideline Legal Framework Remedial Education Treatment Centres* published in January 2011, there is a passage about assessing the ability to give informed consent. This is based on the measures for deciding the ability to give informed consent, according to Appelbaum and Grisso.[10] This is based on the ability to:

- make a choice and to express this
- understand information
- appreciate the situation
- rationally make use of the details.

There is no cut-off score. If one of the above criteria is insufficient, then this indicates the inability to give informed consent.

### 2.4.1 Assessing informed sexual consent

There have been initiatives taken to develop instruments to determine the ability to give informed sexual consent in people with an intellectual disability. The YAI Resource Center in New York has developed the YAI-Tool for Assessing Informed Sexual Consent. This instrument is meant to measure the ability to give informed sexual consent and to assess in which areas a person with an intellectual disability possibly needs further schooling or training regarding sexuality.

Nora J. Baladarian from the United States has developed the FACTS; an interview instrument to test the ability to give informed consent in adults with an intellectual disability, with regard to sexual relationships, by way of making an inventory of the type and consequences of specific sexual acts.

## 2.5 Prevalence of sexual abuse in people with an intellectual disability

International research shows that sexual abuse frequently occurs.[11, 12, 13, 14] Results from research in the Netherlands show that 39 per cent of women and 7 per cent of men without a disability have been victims of sexual violence. The percentage of women and men who have suffered rape is respectively 10 per cent and 1 per cent.[15]

Details about the number of criminal cases hardly form an indication of the actual scale of sexual violence. Only a limited number of cases of sexual violence are reported to the police, and the number of convictions is even lower. In 2004 in the Netherlands, 6668 cases of sexual violence were made known to the police, 2687 cases were solved and in 1585 cases a perpetrator was found guilty.[16]

People with an intellectual disability form an especially vulnerable group regarding the risk of sexual abuse and maltreatment. It is stated in international literature that people with an intellectual disability are made victims of sexual abuse three to five times more often than others in the community.[17, 18, 19, 20, 21, 22] Dutch research also shows that people with an intellectual disability run a substantially higher risk of suffering sexual abuse. Results from the research project 'Limited resilience' by van Berlo and colleagues show that of the people with an intellectual disability, 61 per cent of women and 23 per cent of men have experienced sexual violence in their lives. The sexual violence which they report varies from being touched in an offensive way to rape. In the case of rape, this is reported by 23 per cent of women and 7 per cent of men with an intellectual disability.[23]

Parents, relatives and professionals who are involved with the client with an intellectual disability in this research project report considerably lower percentages. It is concluded that they are often not aware of the situations of sexual abuse. This could also explain that the victims in the research project are mainly people with a mild or moderate intellectual disability. Those with a more severe intellectual disability are dependent on their environment in regard to disclosing the sexual abuse. In diverse publications it is stated that 40 per cent of people with an intellectual disability are made victim of abuse and/or maltreatment before the age of 18.[24] Finally, it is also known that the abuse of people with a disability (due to their continuing dependence on third parties) often lasts for a longer period of time than for people without a disability.[25]

### 2.5.1 Surrounded by care but still not safe

In 2012, the Samson Commission published the results of its research into sexual abuse of children who had been placed out of their homes by the government in the Netherlands: *Surrounded by care, but still not safe.*[26] This shows that children in residential youth care institutions become victims of sexual abuse three to four times more often than average Dutch children.

The Samson Commission conducted specific research into the prevalence of sexual abuse in children with a mild intellectual disability in the Dutch Child Welfare Authority (youth care, childcare).[27] This research was exclusively conducted by intermediaries. On the basis of their observations, children with a mild intellectual disability appear to be three times more often victim of sexual abuse as children without an intellectual disability in the residential child care authority. In concrete terms this means that more than 9.7 of the 1000 children with a mild intellectual disability reported being sexually abused with physical contact in 2010. It is important to mention that cases of sexual abuse previous to the placement in a youth care institution were not included in these figures.

In a research project regarding children with an intellectual disability in a residential home, in which the clients themselves were interviewed, the figures found were 65 per cent for girls and 26 per cent for boys.[28]

International literature shows that children with a (mild) intellectual disability, outside residential homes, also run a higher risk of becoming a victim of sexual abuse.[29, 30] Above all there is a larger chance that people with an intellectual disability will be chronically abused. Classen, Palesh and Aggarwal name alcohol and drug use, psychological issues, interpersonal problems and feelings of shame, guilt and powerlessness as factors which are connected to re-victimisation.[31] It is unclear to what extent these factors are the cause or the effect of re-victimisation and what role the intellectual disability plays in the situation. It is clear, however, that this is a large-scale problem, which frequently confronts practitioners in the care and support of people with an intellectual disability.

### 2.5.2 Perpetrators of sexual abuse

Perpetrators of sexual abuse are usually men, also in the case of male victims. In most cases, the perpetrator is well known to the victim.[32, 33, 34, 35, 36, 37] Research by Samson shows that in 67 per cent of the cases the perpetrators were other youths who were staying in the same care home as the victim. In the 'Limited resilience' study it becomes clear that in a quarter of women with an intellectual disability the sexual violence took place in the care home; this applies to 8 per cent of male victims.[38] International research states that the perpetrator is a professional caregiver in 25 per cent of cases of abuses of people with an intellectual disability.[39] The care relationship is risk heightening due to the dependence aspect. There is also a greater danger of crossing boundaries in care situations which involve physical touch.

Perpetrators are mostly men, both in the case of female and male victims. In approximately half of the cases this concerns other clients who also have a history of abuse and are often admitted to the care home due to this.[40] In 'Limited resilience' from 2011, it is shown that 17 per cent of women with an intellectual disability name their partner as the perpetrator of sexual abuse.[41] It is stated that it is difficult to determine general characteristics of professional caregivers who perpetrate sexual abuse. Where the Samson Commission looked at perpetrators who have been prosecuted and whose cases are pending, it is stated that these are usually native men of average to above-average intelligence. In a quarter of cases the perpetrator has a psychiatric disorder. Their self-image is usually low. About a third of the perpetrators were neglected, maltreated or abused in their youth; in half of cases the perpetrators is married or has been married.

It must be said that these findings cannot be generalised for all perpetrators, as this only concerns those who were prosecuted and/or whose cases are pending.

## 2.6 An explanation of the prevalence of sexual abuse in people with an intellectual disability

Why is it that people with an intellectual disability are more often sexually abused than those of average intelligence? We apply the integrated ecological theory of Dick Sobsey to answer this question.[42] Sobsey is a Canadian professor in the field of people with an intellectual disability and sexual abuse and maltreatment. He published his model in 1999 in his book *Violence and Abuse in the Lives of People with Disabilities: The End of Silent Acceptance?* The model has lost none of its actuality and continues to be used worldwide as a foundation.

The strength of this model lies in the fact that the explanation of the high prevalence figures has revealed that the intellectual disability of people only plays a marginal role. An accumulation of risk factors is present, created by the way in which care is organised. Additionally, social and cultural factors play a role.

The Sobsey model focuses on the interaction of four systems (Figure 2.1). This concerns the characteristics of the potential victim, the potential perpetrator, the characteristics of the immediate social environment and that of the wider society and culture. The four systems influence one another. The more risk factors are present in the various systems, the greater the chance of abuse and maltreatment. It is important here to realise that characteristics which are usually attributed to the intellectual disability are largely influenced by the social environment and not caused by the intellectual disability itself. It is important to acknowledge that, when a large emphasis lies on the characteristic of the potential victim in the explanation of sexual abuse and maltreatment, this can amount to 'blaming the victim'. This seems to be the case in many policy notes.

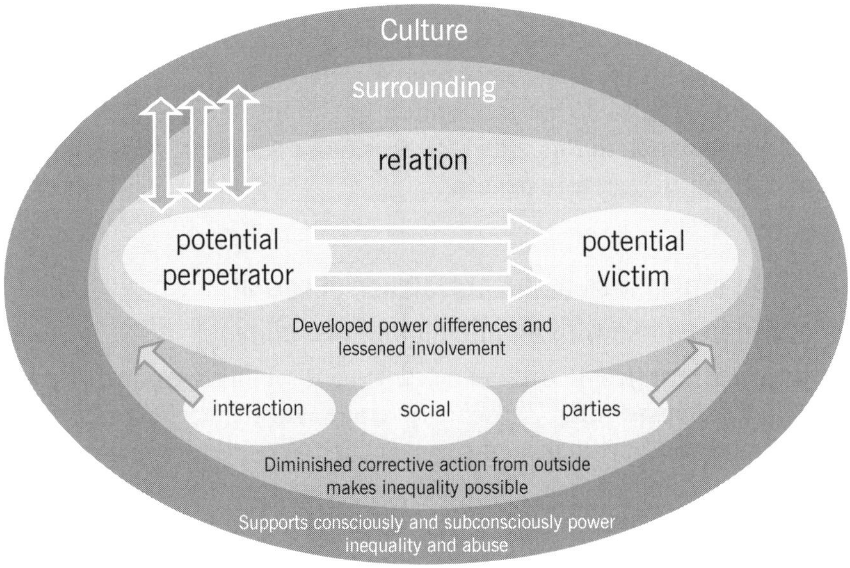


*Figure 2.1 The integrated ecological theory of Sobsey*

As we know, sexual abuse and maltreatment nearly always take place in relationships of dependency. Dependency makes people vulnerable to becoming victim of power abuse and violence in all sorts of situations. A crucial factor in people with an intellectual disability is that they are largely continuously dependant on people around them. Due to the fact that people with an intellectual disability have to undergo so many dependent relationships with often relative strangers, they are primarily educated to adapt to the expectations of others. They learn to be obedient instead of independent, resilient and critical regarding (the intentions of) other people.

Furthermore, many people with an intellectual disability are also dependent on others for physical care. People who need a lot of care learn that their body is not their own, due to the frequency of touch and the many different caregivers who provide the care.[43] Confusion can arise about functional and affective touch and the boundary between desirable and non-desirable touch is difficult to determine. On the grounds of their past history, in which the body has been 'dispossessed', there is often a different understanding of intimacy, physicality and sexuality. People with an intellectual disability will therefore not always know that what has happened to them can be regarded as sexual abuse.

In this situation it can be simpler for the perpetrator to use certain tactics, such as bribery, threats and manipulation. People with an intellectual disability often have limited insight and are less able to see through manipulation. Due to a lack of adequate sexual education and information about their rights, their knowledge of how to act in undesirable situations is often non-existent. People with a disability are also easy victims due to the fact that their disability often limits their ability to communicate and they are therefore less well understood when they attempt to report abuse.[44, 45, 46] Furthermore, a negative sense of self, negative physical image and problems with social emotional development are also considered to be risk factors.[47, 48, 49]

Alongside risk factors which concern the victim there are, as Sobsey also states in his theory, situational and social factors which can heighten the risks. For example, situations in which people live or work together closely and where there are clear power differences, situations in which women are under-represented, and traditional communities in which conservative opinions about male and female behaviour and sexuality prevail.[50, 51, 52, 53]

For people with an intellectual disability who live in a residential care home, social isolation often occurs, as does a lack of social control.[54] Due to this isolation they often have limited opportunity to experience the 'conventional' social forms which exist in the community.[55] Above all, the chance is greater that a person will come into contact with others who have been victims – and/or perpetrators – of sexual abuse. There is therefore an increased chance of a person (again) becoming a victim of sexual abuse.

## 2.7 The implications of sexual abuse in people with an intellectual disability

Sexual abuse does not only affect the victim, but also has a large impact on the people around them. In order to understand the implications of sexual abuse for a child with an intellectual disability, it is essential to be aware of the influence of having a child with an intellectual disability. There is a special dynamic within families with a child with an intellectual disability. Being the parent of such a child gives rise to confusing feelings. The parents love their child and are happy with their child, but at the same time they would have liked things to be different. They can have feelings of fear, shame and/or resistance, which in turn lead to feelings of guilt. Parents can ask themselves: Why did this happen to us? Surely my child didn't deserve this? What does the future hold? The birth of a child with a disability can come as a shock, and feel like an experience of loss.

### 2.7.1 Parents

There is a special dynamic surrounding the vulnerability of the child with an intellectual disability. All parents want to protect their children against the evil in the world. This is even more strongly developed in parents with a child with a disability. These parents are confronted by the vulnerability of their child each and every day. It is often more difficult to let go of their child and to see their child as a separate person with their own feelings and emotions.

Standard developmental processes such as separation and individuality are more limited. There is often the feeling of a merged existence, in that parents can experience the abuse as something which has not only been done to their child, but also directly to themselves. Parents of abused children with an intellectual disability frequently express the feeling of having been sexually abused themselves. Their reactions are therefore even more intense. All parents who are confronted by the sexual abuse of their child experience intense feelings of disbelief, upset and anger. A reaction which is often observed is that parents feel guilty about the sexual abuse of their child. They think that they should have recognised that the abuse was taking place and realised what was happening to their child.[56] They believe they should have protected their child and the feeling that they failed in doing so creates shame and sadness. These feelings of guilt can evolve into the belief that they aren't a good mother or father. It is also possible that parents have difficulty in believing their child. It is important to inform parents about the fact that children seldom lie about sexual abuse.

The issue of mortality also plays a role for parents of children with an intellectual disability. They are faced with questions and fears such as: What will happen when we aren't there anymore? Who will look after my child then? If this happens while I'm alive then what will happen when I'm not there to protect them?

### 2.7.2 Accumulated powerlessness

In the case of sexual abuse in children with an intellectual disability, parents can experience accumulated powerlessness.[57] In the first place, parents have given birth to a child with a disability. Although many parents do not dare to express this, deep inside they can see it as a failure. They have not succeeded in creating a healthy child and they could not do anything about it; the first feeling of powerlessness is born.

If the child is placed out of the home, the second feeling of powerlessness can be the fact that the parents cannot bring up their child themselves. The abuse of the child prompts many feelings of powerlessness. The way in which the healthcare organisation or police and justice system handles the situation can increase the feeling of powerlessness in parents. It goes without saying that the reaction of the parents to the abuse of their child is affected and intensified by the accumulated powerlessness described here.

Furthermore, the discovery that the child has been sexually abused can trigger many painful feelings and memories in parents who have experienced sexual abuse themselves. Old defence mechanisms in the parent can arise, such as distancing themselves from the situation in order to avoid or ignore the unbearable feelings.[58] The consequence can be that parents deny or trivialise the fact that abuse has taken place.

## 2.8 The well-known perpetrator

Perpetrators of sexual abuse in people with an intellectual disability are generally known to the victim.[59, 60, 61, 62] Due to the dependency of many people with an intellectual disability, there is a high chance that the perpetrator is also known to the parents and/or professional caregivers. The discovery that the abuse has been perpetrated by someone who was trusted can cause intense feelings of anger, guilt, denial and disbelief. Parents and professional caregivers can be confused about the fact that they could have been so wrong about people they thought they knew. This disturbs their basis of trust in the world.[63]

If the perpetrator is one of the parents or professional caregivers, those involved will feel even more hurt and betrayed. The feeling of certainty is lost and relationships are dramatically disturbed. These processes within the family and team of healthcare professionals also affect the larger social system. Sides often form, and ties with family, friends and colleagues come under pressure and can become a minefield. This process of splitting is described in other places in this book (see Sections 2.2.1 and 9.1.6).

## 2.9 Consequences of sexual abuse in victims with an intellectual disability

People who have been confronted by sexual abuse usually feel lonely, abandoned, guilty, damaged and scared. They experience powerlessness and have the feeling that the obviousness and justice of life have been lost. Their trust in other people has been seriously damaged.

If their world has been damaged in this way, there is a large chance that stress reactions will occur. These reactions are healthy and normal reactions to abnormal and unhealthy incidents. The seriousness and scale of the consequences of sexual abuse are dependent on a number of factors, which are shown in Box 2.2.

Sexual abuse has the same consequences in people with an intellectual disability as in people without an intellectual disability. The consequences can, however, be made worse by the way in which help is organised for a person with an intellectual disability. It is clear that the factors which increase the seriousness of the consequences of sexual abuse (a known perpetrator and long-term sexual abuse) often apply in the case of a person with an intellectual disability. Above all, people with an intellectual disability are largely dependent on the reactions and support of significant others and the way in which they cope with the sexual abuse. In practice, there appears to be a great lack in the ability to actually create a safe environment and provide adequate support after sexual abuse. See the text about coping with trauma in people with an intellectual disability (Section 4.5).

## Box 2.2 Factors which determine the seriousness of sexual abuse

- *The relationship of the victim with the perpetrator*
  The stronger the attachment, the greater the risk of a trauma. There is also a greater chance that the capability of the victim to trust another person is damaged. These victims tend to blame themselves for the abuse more than people who have been abused by strangers.
- *The seriousness and length of the sexual abuse*
  A sexual activity without physical contact appears to be less traumatic. The longer the period of time in which the abuse takes place, the higher the risk of damaging consequences. The more violence is used, the more serious the consequences are.[64]
- *The age (and the developmental level) of the victim*
  The younger the victim, the more serious the consequences. Sexual abuse affects the development of the brain of the victim; there are therefore (especially) damaging consequences in the case of victims who are too young to remember the abuse.[65]
- *The reaction of the surroundings after the sexual abuse*
  If a victim is not believed, or is blamed or ignored, this will increase the chance of psychological problems. A lack of supportive adults increases the feelings of loneliness, helplessness and worthlessness and this has a negative effect on the seriousness of the trauma. Above all, the symptoms often worsen if victims are silent for years about their experiences and do not receive help straightaway.[66]

## 2.10 Victims of sexual abuse and sexually inappropriate behaviour

People who have been abused can start demonstrating sexually inappropriate behaviour themselves. This usually concerns reactive behaviour as a consequence of the sexual abuse which they have suffered. People demonstrating this behaviour obviously require clear and consequent boundaries. In addition, it is important to understand how the behaviour started and the implications this has for this client, so that adequate behaviour alternatives can be offered. See the various exercises in Chapter 10.

---

It is extremely important that the focus during treatment is not on 'perpetrator behaviour' and the corresponding interventions. Experience teaches that after adequate trauma treatment this behaviour soon ceases.

---

## 2.11 Sexual education for people who have been sexually abused

People with an intellectual disability who have been sexually abused often receive sexual education as a reaction to what has happened. It is important to realise that, by doing so, clients implicitly receive the message that there is a relationship between the knowledge which they have about sexuality and the fact that someone has abused them. This does not seem to coincide with the reality of the situation and puts the responsibility for the abuse in the wrong place. It is therefore recommended not to apply standard sexual education as an intervention after sexual abuse, but to make it a preventative part of the education and support.

Victims often wrestle with questions concerning sexuality after sexual abuse. If the perpetrator is of the same sex as the victim, doubts about sexual preference can arise. Additionally, questions arise about issues such as the relationship between aggression and sexuality, the relationship between sexuality and love and between power, love and sex, and also the relationship between arousal, will and responsibility. These questions are not addressed in standard educational material.

The tone of the standard educational material does not seem to match the perception and experience of victims.[67] It is recommended to pay attention to these issues by using a specialised curriculum. This should take place after trauma treatment, for example in the last phase of treatment.[68] Here the client can learn to talk about the norms and values, boundaries and desires of a physical, intimate and sexual nature, under the guidance of the therapist, together with the parent/guardian or professional caregiver. Alternative behaviour should also be suggested. An advantage of this method is that, at the same time, the isolation of the victim regarding this issue is broken and, due to the examples of behaviour, the caregiver will receive tools with which to talk to the client about this subject in daily life. In this way, not only coping with the past is addressed, but important preventative conditions can also be created for the future.

## SUMMARY

National and international research states that sexual abuse is a large-scale problem worldwide. Sexual abuse occurs more often in people with an intellectual disability than in those without an intellectual disability. The abuse creates different dynamics within a family and within the wider system of a person with an intellectual disability. Sexual abuse gives rise to feelings of powerlessness in the victim and in the surrounding social environment. In the case of parents of a child with an intellectual disability, accumulated powerlessness is often seen. This is the build-up of the feelings of helplessness as the result of having a child with an intellectual disability, of having to witness how the child cannot keep up in the world, of (partly) having to let others care for the child and then, added to this, the incident(s) of sexual abuse. The way in which the sexual abuse situation is handled by the healthcare organisation involved or by the police and the justice system can increase the feelings of powerlessness in the parents.

These dynamics require a specific approach by the healthcare professionals involved. It is important that there is awareness of the fact that the vulnerability of the victim is not a characteristic which results purely from having an intellectual disability. A one-sided emphasis on the disability as cause of the abuse can lead to 'blaming the victim'. In the explanation of the high prevalence of sexual abuse in people with an intellectual disability, attention must be paid to the situational and social factors which play a role in this issue. Here lies an important point of attention for the prevention of sexual abuse of people with an intellectual disability.

## Chapter 3

# THE LEGAL FRAMEWORK IN CASES OF SEXUAL ABUSE OF PEOPLE WITH AN INTELLECTUAL DISABILITY

### Introduction

Healthcare professionals involved in the care of people with an intellectual disability have a special responsibility for the safety of their clients. Despite all preventative measures, they are unfortunately often confronted by situations involving (suspected) sexual abuse. Healthcare professionals may encounter sexual abuse in various ways. The victim and perpetrator may be clients, but also employees, volunteers or interns. The abuse can involve someone well known to the client, such as a family member or a friend. Sexual abuse can be disclosed by the victim or those in their immediate environment or discovered by coincidence, but it can also come to light after investigating indirect signs. Only in a few cases is the perpetrator caught in the act.

The (suspected) victim must be protected, but also the (suspected) perpetrator must be treated carefully. The situation can be very complicated and great care must be taken in dealing with it. In situations of (suspected) sexual abuse there is a special dynamic, in which emotions, loyalty, individual perception, accusations and the safety of clients play a large role. Clear policy regarding sexual abuse, based on a clear vision in this area, provides a focus in this complex dynamic and is essential for adequate action of healthcare professionals in situations of (suspected) sexual abuse.

In this chapter, attention is paid to the rights and obligations which apply in dealing with suspicions of sexual abuse. There is attention given to the reporting code for calamities and sexual abuse at the Inspection for Healthcare,[1] the reporting code for domestic violence and child abuse and the obligation for using sexual abuse protocols. In addition, relevant legal articles are described in short. The possibilities for a legal course of action are also addressed, including making a report and statement to the police. There is specific focus on talking about sexual abuse with a suspected victim – the role of the minimum fact interview is often essential for this. Finally, guidelines are provided for dealing with the media in situations of sexual abuse.

## 3.1 Reporting obligation, reporting code and sexual abuse protocol

Since the change in the Dutch Quality Act for healthcare institutions,[2] there is a legal requirement to report calamities and sexual abuse to the Dutch Healthcare Inspectorate. Care organisations are also obliged to investigate the reports and to report this to the inspection service. The Dutch Healthcare Inspectorate states that it is compulsory to follow a protocol in suspicions of sexual abuse in *It's not allowed…it's never allowed.*[3] An adequate protocol is based on a vision and is clearly and concretely formulated: tasks and responsibilities are clearly described. Not only employees, but also clients and their legal representatives must be aware of the content of the protocol. Adhering to a protocol prevents people acting on the basis of their emotions and ensures that situations can be investigated and dealt with objectively.

Most care institutions have described their vision on sexual abuse and the prevention of such in a protocol, focusing on dealing with situations of sexual abuse. There is, however, still much to be improved regarding the implementation and the embedding of such vision and policy documents in organisations. This is an important task for the employee concerned with sexuality issues, and for policy employees and managers. It has become apparent in various organisations that the implementation can be more adequately conducted when time and materials are provided. It is also essential that managers give the subject high priority and consciously consider it to be their personal responsibility to address it properly.

### 3.1.1 Law reporting code domestic violence and child abuse

Alongside the requirements of the Dutch Healthcare Inspectorate, it has been compulsory in the Netherlands since 2013 for organisations and independent professionals (including healthcare, education, childcare, youth care and social support) to use a reporting code for domestic violence and child abuse – including sexual abuse.

This means that it is compulsory for healthcare professionals to report (suspected) sexual abuse within the organisation. This obligation prevents an employee ignoring a suspicion based on uncertainty, collegial feelings or fear of consequences. It also prevents signs of sexual abuse being interpreted by an individual employee and being dealt with according to their own personal insight and interests. This means that suspicions of sexual abuse come to light faster and it is possible to investigate concerns and signs at an early stage and (if necessary) to act adequately.

The Mandatory Reporting Code Act does not include a reporting code outside the organisation. The decision to report suspicions of (child) abuse by others than professionals to the AMK (Dutch Advice and Reporting Centre for Child Abuse) or SHG (Domestic Violence Advice and Support Centre) is up to the professional and the care provider where this person works.

There is a special legal notice about external reports in the Child Welfare Act (Jeugdzorgwet); this is about situations in which suspicions of child abuse concern healthcare professionals. The legal notice states that in such cases, it is compulsory to file a report with the Children's Welfare Office (Bureau Jeugdzorg).[4]

## 3.2 Laws and regulations

Professionals within the healthcare service for people with an intellectual disability have to work with various laws and regulations (alongside reporting obligation, reporting codes and protocols). These sometimes seem to give contradictory directions, and a 'conflict of duties' can arise for healthcare professionals when reporting (suspected) sexual abuse. This conflict can be between the obligation to ensure the safety of a client and the need to adhere to professional confidentiality and/or privacy law regulations. Another conflict can arise between the obligation to inform parents and/or other authorities in a client's life and the obligation not to do so if and when informing others would endanger the client.

The most important laws and regulations in situations of sexual abuse are described in this section, without the intention of providing a complete overview of information. As a source of information we have used the Netherlands Association for Disability Care and the Knowledge Place for Disability Care: Directing the approach to sexual abuse.[5]

### 3.2.1 Who has to give permission?

The Medical Treatment Contracts Act (WGBO) includes a special regulation of the control of investigation or treatment, concerning diagnostic research, conducting a minimum fact interview and making a report or statement to the police by care providers. The regulation groups people into three age groups.

#### *Children under 12 years of age*

For investigation and treatment of a child under 12 years of age, permission is required from the legal representative(s) of the child. They decide about research and/or treatment. The process can be conducted without permission from the parents or guardian if and when this is necessary in order to prevent serious disadvantage for the client, if the client – also after the refusal of the representatives of the child to give permission – continues to desire the process after proper consideration.[6]

This means that in situations in which there are great concerns about safety, investigations can be conducted in the interest of the client, without permission from the legal representatives. This can be the case, for example, if there are suspicions of sexual abuse possibly occurring within the family.

### *Children between 12 and 15 years of age*

In this age group, both the permission of the child and that of the authoritative party are required. The process can be conducted without the permission of the authoritative party if and when this is deemed necessary to prevent serious disadvantage for the client, and if the client – also after the refusal of the representatives of the child to give permission – continues to desire the process after proper consideration.[7]

This means that in cases in which the parents and their child are not in agreement, the practitioner should follow the opinion of the child. The safety and the interests of the child should always be the priority. In adherence to these rights of the child, the healthcare professional should take the involvement of the parents into account.

### *Adolescents of 16 and 17 years of age*

An underaged client who has reached the age of 16 is (if able to give consent) authorised to make an agreement regarding themselves. In addition they are also able to conduct legal actions which are connected to the agreement. This means that a client can follow a diagnostic course of action, a minimum fact interview or give a report or statement, without the permission of parents.[8]

### *Clients who are unable to give consent*

Clients who are not able to give consent are represented by their parents or guardians.[9] They are authorised to give permission for investigations and treatment and also practise the other patient's rights for the client. It is possible to deviate from this rule if desired by the care of a good healthcare professional.[10] The healthcare professional can then act outside of the legal representatives. This can be necessary if the safety of the client is at stake.

## 3.2.2 In which cases is permission necessary?

In the case of (suspected) sexual abuse, consultation between the professionals involved is required. For discussion within the organisation, with a knowledgeable colleague or special task employee on sexuality within the organisation, permission from the child or the parent(s) for providing these details is not necessary. This also applies to any advice sought from the Child Welfare Office or the Advice and Reporting Centre for Child Abuse (AMK) or the police, if the client details are kept anonymous. According to the Child Welfare Act, a professional is permitted to provide personal information about the child or their parent(s) if and when the AMK requests this – this can also be possible without permission of the child or the parent(s).

For reporting or discussing with someone outside the organisation where one is working (and in which the details about the client and/or parent(s) are provided), permission is necessary. The regulations are not uniform. The Personal Data Protection Act states that, from 16 years of age, a client must give a professional permission for giving their details to others (whether or not in the form of a report). The Child Welfare Office Act and the WGBO give a client this right from the age of 12. If this concerns a client up to 16 years of age who lives at home, it is compulsory to talk to the parent(s) because usually not only details about the child are given, but also about the parent(s).

On the grounds of the WGBO, it is possible to give information to third parties about a client or the network without permission from a client or legal representative(s).[11] This is, however, only permitted if it is deemed necessary in order to stop the sexual abuse, and it is the only available way to achieve this.

### 3.2.3 Building dossiers and the right to access

All information which is important for the treatment of the client should be recorded in the client dossier, including information regarding (a suspicion of) sexual abuse. A record should be kept in this dossier of which signs indicated a suspicion of sexual abuse, the reaction to this and which arguments have led to a report and/or statement. The report of a minimum fact interview should be kept in the client dossier. Because this concerns an investigation, conducted by a professional, this is preferably kept in the part of the dossier which is meant for behavioural science diagnostics.

According to the Dutch Personal Data Protection Act, reports of sexual incidents are confidential information. From the perspective of privacy, it is in principle not permitted to mention the name of the victim in the dossier of the perpetrator and vice versa. From the perspective of safety and good healthcare, it is actually necessary to be aware of these details. Clients with an intellectual disability are often not able to provide this information themselves. Above all, healthcare professionals often change jobs and do not always know what has happened in the life history of the client.

Recording information in the dossier is necessary to prevent a victim in the same institution (or in a following institution) finding themselves in a situation in which they are once again, living with a perpetrator from the past, or running into one another at a bus stop or in a workplace. Safety should be the priority here above privacy!

### *Right to access information*

A client and their authorities have the right to access dossier papers, including reports of diagnostics and minimum fact interviews. A request for access to the dossier does not have to be granted, insofar as this is necessary in the interest of the protection of the personal life of the other person.[12] It should be considered that, if authoritative parties are still to be heard by the police, it is important that they have not (yet) read the report of the minimum fact interview. This prevents contamination of their story.

According to the WGBO, parents have the right to access the dossier of their child who is under 16 years of age. This is also applicable when this contains details which the child has shared in the trust that their parents will not be told about them. The WGBO offers the professional the possibility of not giving permission for the parents to access these details on the grounds of the following legal notice:

> If and when the professional, upon receiving information about the patient or upon inspection or copy of the documents provided, is not able to provide good professional care, he may omit doing so.[13]

### 3.2.4 Information obligation

For clients under the age of 12 years old, and for clients unable to give informed consent, authoritative parties have the right to information about the investigation and treatment. The child also has their own right to information, adapted to their ability for comprehension.[14] The law states that the authoritative parent informs the parent which is not authoritative about serious situations regarding the under-aged child.[15]

Not only authoritative parties, but also non-authoritative parties have the right to be informed about cases that would be provided to authoritative parents. This is not the case if the interests of the child are contradictory to providing information. The juridical starting point is that the non-authoritative parent must ask for information (has to be active in doing so) and that the information must be provided, unless the situation is considered to be exceptional. Informing parents can be left out of consideration in the interests of providing good healthcare support; for example, in cases in which confidentiality is necessary for the care of the child.

### 3.2.5 Professional confidentiality and the reporting code

Professional confidentiality is stated in various legal notices,[16] professional codes and behavioural rules of professional groups. Professional confidentiality includes the pledge of secrecy and the right to refuse to give evidence.

The pledge of secrecy means that a healthcare professional does not say anything about the case unless the patient gives permission for him or her to talk. The pledge of secrecy does not apply to other professionals who are directly involved in the implementattion of the case agreement.

The Child Welfare Act contains a clear reporting right: every practitioner with a professional confidentiality or other pledge to secrecy has the right to report suspicions of child abuse to the AMK, if necessary without the permission of the child or parent(s).[17] There are possible situations in which healthcare professionals break secrecy pledge because a different interest, such as safety, is more significant. Breaking the pledge to secrecy is not a criminal offence if it is possible to successfully appeal to circumstances beyond one's control (see Box 3.1).[18]

**Box 3.1 Circumstances beyond one's control**

According to the justice system and literature, the following five questions must be considered in order to define whether the circumstances are beyond one's control:

1. Which aim do I want to achieve by talking to someone else?
2. Is there a different possibility in order to achieve this aim, without having to break my professional confidentiality?
3. Why is it not possible to ask for or receive permission?
4. Are the interests of the client whom I wish to help by talking so serious that they outweigh the interests of the client (and parents) if I keep quiet?
5. If I decide to talk, to whom must I provide information so that the client can be helped?

### 3.2.6 The right to refuse to give evidence

The right to refuse to give evidence refers to the right to remain silent about certain details concerning the patient.[19] The right to refuse to give evidence also applies with regard to the judge. Due to the fact that the information which is given to police can also be used by the judge, the right to refuse to give evidence can also be exercised towards the police.

If a healthcare professional is called as a witness in a criminal case, they are obliged to appear, but can appeal to their (secondary) right to refuse to give evidence. The judge decides if this appeal can be honoured. If the judge rejects the appeal then the healthcare professional is obliged to talk. People with a secondary professional confidentiality also have a secondary right to refuse to give evidence.[20, 21]

The interests of the client must be considered when making an appeal for the right to refuse to give evidence. The interests of the client are often benefited when the healthcare professional does give evidence so in these cases it may not be appropriate to hide behind the right to refuse to give evidence.

## 3.3 Minimum fact interviews

An important instrument in dealing with suspicions of sexual abuse is the minimum fact interview. A minimum fact interview is a healthcare support conversation which aims, in a methodical way, to clarify unclear signs which could indicate sexual abuse and/or maltreatment. Conducting a minimum fact interview can strengthen the legal position of people with an intellectual disability by preventing people talking in a suggestive and unprofessional manner about the suspicions. According to the guidelines of the Society for Disability Care in the Netherlands (VGN), many care institutions that work with people with intellectual disabilities include the minimum fact interview in their protocol on (suspected) sexual abuse. A minimum fact interview is not meant to determine whether or not sexual abuse took place – deciding about that is the task of the police and justice system.

A minimum fact interview is only to be conducted by professionals who have been educated to do so. In the minimum fact interview method, the professional uses objective and neutral questioning with the focus on gathering information, in which they take into account a possible police and/or legal course of action. The minimum fact interview should be a part of a sexual abuse protocol and is nowadays part of a growing number of care providers' co-operation agreements.

When a minimum fact interview is conducted with a client, it is important to consider the use of the SOS handbook carefully. The SOS programme can be started at the moment of disclosure or discovery of a situation of sexual abuse, preferably soon after the minimum fact interview. A minimum fact interview is not necessary in the case of a clear disclosure or if someone is caught in the act. Immediate consultation with the police is then emphatically advised.

## 3.4 Statement or report to the police

Many doubts or differences in opinion about the credibility of the story play a role in situations of (suspected) sexual abuse. Determining the truth about the (suspicion of) sexual abuse is not a task for the healthcare professionals. In the case of (suspected) sexual abuse it is always, at the earliest stage possible, advisable to (informally) talk to the police, preferably in the area in which the sexual abuse took place. Talking to the police at an early stage makes it possible to start working together straightaway, to co-ordinate efforts and to consider the optimal approach together. This helps to prevent unintentional damage towards the client and the police investigation.

If possible, it is advisable to make decisions about filing a report or statement with the police in close consultation with the suspected victim and their parents/guardians (see Box 3.2). The difference between a report and a statement is that a report only leads to registration. Information can be included in other possible investigations or in future statements. In extremely serious cases it is possible that the police will take up the case officially and conduct an investigation. A statement leads to a police investigation and prosecution.

## Box 3.2 Statement versus report

The following points are important in deciding whether to make a statement or a report:[22]

- It is often advised not to make a police statement in the case of victims with an intellectual disability due to the fear that the hearing will be too much of a burden for them. Experience teaches that a police interview can actually be the beginning of the coping process for the clients, if the hearing is conducted well.[23] Depending on the complexity of the situation, specially trained police agents and external experts from the hearing pool are available to conduct the hearing. Clients seldom experience the hearing as an extra burden.
- Making a statement involves the question of finding the perpetrator. Clients can be transferred to a safe place for a long period. This can also serve the interests of the care institution and the whole community.
- The statement process is often lengthy. Due to the fact that most cases of sexual abuse are hard to prove, they do not often result in a court case. If a case does result in a court case it often ends in an acquittal on the grounds of too little evidence. This must, however, never be used as a reason not to make a statement.

At the same time, it is important to discuss the expectations of a client and their system and to give them honest information about the course of action of the police and the justice system.

---

Reports and statements of (suspected) sexual abuse can be made by anyone who is aware of the situation or has a suspicion of the situation. Who actually makes the statement or report depends on the situation and should (if possible) be decided after discussion with the client, authoritative party and the police. It is advised that the wishes of the client are followed as far as possible.

At the same time, it is important to realise that for people with an intellectual disability (and also for those without a disability) it is difficult to imagine something which they do not know. Healthcare support institutions have their own responsibility concerning making a statement or a report: the safety of their clients and possibly also other employees is always the priority! If the victim and their legal representatives decide not to make a statement or a report, the organisation (definitely in the case of a serious crime) has a moral duty to do so.

In many cases of sexual abuse of people with an intellectual disability it is advised to let the manager of the healthcare organisation concerned make the statement. A person who makes a statement cannot be heard as a witness. If a healthcare institution makes a statement, then those directly involved can still act as a witness, if the manager has made the statement. This is of great importance in cases of (suspected) sexual abuse, in which evidence is already so problematic!

### *Studio interview*

If the decision is made to file a complaint with the police, an interview with witnesses (parents, caregivers) and the alleged victim will follow (see Section 3.4.2). The normal course of action is that the police prepare the client and their parents and legal representatives for the interview. It is sometimes recommended to ask a professional involved in the situation to carry out the preparation, as they can take into account the abilities and disabilities of the client.

According to the directions for investigation and prosecution regarding sexual abuse, in cases of sexual crimes involving under-aged people with an intellectual disability and people with a cognitive functioning disorder (both witnesses and declarants), the interview is conducted by specially trained police agents. This takes place in a special audio visual studio.[24] Due to the complexity of such an interview, external experts (specialised in interviewing people with an intellectual disability) have an important advisory role. If required due to the complexity of the disability, the police can ask the justice officer for permission to use specialists who are certified experts in this area (see Chapter 10, Information sheet: Studio hearing).

When the police have completed the investigation and found sufficient evidence against the accused, the dossier is sent to the officer of justice, who decides whether or not a court case will be held.

### 3.4.1 Support in making the statement

If a statement of sexual abuse is made, it is of great importance that a client is carefully supported in doing so. It is advisable to name one or two contact persons. In the choice of caregivers it is important to take into account the wishes of the victim as much as possible.

It is also important to be aware that supporting a victim during the process of making a statement can be very intense. Before the actual statement, an informative discussion takes place with the police. In this discussion the police describe what making a statement involves and explain the process. It is advisable to weigh up the advantages this discussion will have for the client themselves and whether it might be preferable to let the client only attend the studio hearing. The reason for this lies in the fact that the informative discussion is often not conducted by specialised police officials who have been educated to work with this group of people. At the time of the informative discussion it is often not clear that that is necessary. The consequence is that it can be difficult to take into account the conversational level of the client during the discussion and therefore it can be unintentionally disturbing for the rest of the procedure. The chance of influencing the investigation increases if the client is spoken to during this discussion (whether this is in a suitable way for the client's conversational level or not).

After the informative discussion, if desired, an appointment is made for the actual statement. Make clear agreements about who the contact person is for the police and how, when and by whom the information is communicated to the client, their system and the healthcare professionals involved.

If a statement is made, it can be necessary to request the services of a specialised lawyer. In the Dutch legal system, the legal position of victims is not very strong. This is especially the case for people with an intellectual disability. Additionally, a lawyer can be needed if the interests of the client with an intellectual disability contradict the interests of the care institution, or if clients (and/or their authoritative parties) are of the opinion that the care institution has acted in a sloppy or careless manner. A lawyer can also be connected to a criminal case and demand damages (for example, to pay for therapy) and/or a contact ban and/or moving house ban. Moreover, in cases of sexual abuse it is often possible to request damage compensation from the Damage Fund for Violent Crimes.

### Box 3.3 Free legal assistance

Since April 2006, the legal help for victims of sexual crimes is free of charge, under certain conditions. The condition is that a prosecution has been started. There is more information available about this from the National Lawyers' Network Sexual Offence Victims (Landelijk Advocaten Netwerk Zeden Slachtoffers) which focuses on the legal support for victims of sexual crimes.[25] In Alkmaar, Rotterdam and Utrecht, networks of lawyers providing legal support for victims of sexual violence (JOS: Juridische Opvang Slachtoffers seksueel geweld) can also be found.

## 3.4.2 Talking about sexual abuse and the police interview

From the moment that the suspicion of sexual abuse first arises, those involved both inside and outside the organisation need honest and carefully considered information. Taking into account the right to remain silent with regard to a judiciary investigation, all of those involved benefit most from as much openness as possible. However, it is not necessary or desirable to make all details public. It is recommended to decide which information can be communicated to the outside world in consultation with the police. In this way, things which are unclear, speculations and sensational stories can be prevented from occurring.[26]

Talking about abuse with a client with an intellectual disability requires instructions at the point in the process when the possible police interview has yet to take place. It is important to consider the fact that the client, as witness in a criminal case, should be influenced as little as possible. The longer it takes before the police hear the client, the greater the chance of 'contamination' of the story. It is therefore recommended to make clear to the police the importance of the hearing taking place as soon as possible.

---

When the hearing of the client is completed, there is no reason to be reserved in speaking about what has happened. Before that time, caution is advised!

---

If the hearing has yet to take place, it is recommended not to ask questions about facts (who, what, where, when and how) during discussions with the victim and not to ask probing questions about the facts. You can listen to the story which the client tells and emphasise that the client is now safe (if that is actually the case). Furthermore, you can say that it is very good that the client has told their story.

The focus of the discussions with the client, before the studio hearing has taken place, lies mainly on providing psychoeducation about possible after-effects which the client is suffering. Ways in which the client can learn to deal with these symptoms are considered together. In this phase, people have to search for whichever possibilities are available for support and guidance, without contradicting the protocol for (suspected) sexual abuse or endangering the possible police investigation. The content of the SOS programme is adapted according to this issue.

Close collaboration between healthcare professionals and the police during the process is required. The safety and interests of the client are always the deciding factor!

## 3.5 Medical investigation

In the Netherlands, doctors are seldom involved in investigations into (suspected) sexual abuse. In many situations of (suspected) sexual abuse in people with an intellectual disability it is recommended to ask for medical tests to be conducted. To do so, it is important to contact the police as soon as possible, who can then call in a gynaecologist to conduct a sexual test, so that evidence can be taken and stored safely. Tests aimed at determining pregnancy, sexually transmitted diseases (STDs) and internal injuries should be conducted by a specialised gynaecologist, in consultation with the police. Investigations by a forensic doctor are recommended, especially in situations with victims with a severe intellectual disability where finding evidence is problematic. There is a forensic out-patients clinic for child abuse which specialises in this form of investigation.[27] If the abuse took place less than 72 hours ago, traces can best be taken if the clothing of the victim has not been washed, the client has not been to the toilet (keep and bring possible urine and excrement to the investigation), and possible clothes or other objects are kept in paper (definitely not plastic!).

Sometimes abnormalities (such as injuries, infections, STDs and/or pregnancy) are detected, which can support the suspicion of sexual abuse. If no physical indications are found for sexual abuse, this does not mean that it did not take place. Some sexual acts do not cause visible damage and sometimes the abuse took place so long ago that injuries have healed.[28] Medical tests provide evidence that abuse has taken place in less than 10 per cent of people for whom there is a suspicion of having been sexually abused.

## 3.6 Dealing with the media

If there is a suspicion of sexual abuse, particularly when it involves people with an intellectual disability, it can attract large-scale media attention. It is important that care institutions operate proactively with regard to the media, with an open and transparent approach. It is of the utmost importance that the care institution makes sure that parents, relatives and others involved know about what has happened before any media reporting. By providing correct and focused information, a basis of trust can be established with everyone.

Writing a clear press release is often effective with regard to dealing with the media. If organisations refuse to give information to the press, the chance is high that journalists will search for sources themselves and in this way will receive and distribute incomplete and incorrect information. It is important to name a spokesperson within the organisation. All employees must know the name of this spokesperson, so that other colleagues can refer the press to them if they seek contact. Other employees should be instructed, in a positive and friendly manner, to refrain from giving any sort of commentary.

The subject of the media should also be discussed with the client and their system in order to prepare them for sudden contact with the media. It is recommended to prepare a possible reaction together.

Finally, consideration should be given to the way in which other clients and parents might be approached by the media and how they can be prepared for sudden contact with the press.

## SUMMARY

The reporting obligation, reporting codes and the sexual abuse protocol help healthcare professionals act adequately in situations of (suspected) sexual abuse. Due to the fact that in these situations the healthcare, police and justice system are often working in a tense environment, it is important to have a working knowledge of laws and regulations. Professionals in the care of people with an intellectual disability are affected by various laws and regulations on this issue. These sometimes seem to give opposing directions, which can result in a 'conflict of duty' for the healthcare professionals involved. Ultimately, the interests and safety of the client and others is always the main factor in dealing with conflicts of this nature.

According to the guidelines of the disability council, many care institutions which work with people with an intellectual disability have included minimum fact interviews in their protocol for (suspected) sexual abuse. The minimum fact interview is not meant to determine if sexual abuse has occurred. Finding out the truth is the task of the police and justice system. The SOS handbook can be used from the moment at which a situation of sexual abuse is disclosed or discovered. It is important when making a report or statement that, where possible, this is done in consultation with other clients involved in the situation, authoritative parties and the police. Healthcare professionals and care institutions also have their own responsibility: the safety of their clients and others is always the priority.

From the first moment that a suspicion of sexual abuse arises, those involved within and outside the organisation need honest and carefully considered information. All of those involved benefit mostly from openness about the issue, without having to explain everything in detail. Openness is also important in conversations with the client with an intellectual disability about this subject. However, before the police interview has taken place, all of those involved must keep to strict guidelines so as not to negatively influence the police investigation. Close collaboration between healthcare professionals and the police is required for this purpose.

## Chapter 4

# TRAUMA AND COPING WITH TRAUMA

## Introduction

Sexual abuse is a shocking experience which has a serious impact on people's lives. Shocking experiences such as these are also referred to as a traumatic event or as the experience of trauma. What traumatic events all have in common is that they are far removed from the normal human experience and the basic feeling of safety is seriously damaged, either once or repeatedly. Experiencing trauma can have various consequences at a psychological, social and neurobiological level. Coping with trauma can involve stress reactions, which, if they last for a long period of time, can develop into a post-traumatic stress disorder.

For the professional who conducts the SOS programme, it is important to have background information about various issues which can play a role in trauma. This information can help to interpret the behaviour of the client, the parents, relatives and the team of healthcare professionals. Being able to recognise (traumatic) stress reactions in the various age phases plays an important role in psychoeducation in the SOS programme. The practitioner must be aware of issues such as dissociation and secondary traumatic stress.

Coping with traumatic events and associated stress reactions is more difficult for people with an intellectual disability. Due to their life history and cognitive disability, these people have less adequate coping mechanisms to deal with overwhelming circumstances. They are vulnerable to psychological problems in general and there are indications which suggest that they also develop post-traumatic stress disorders sooner than people without a disability.

For this reason it is essential that professionals have specific knowledge about how people with an intellectual disability cope with trauma and associated issues such as disharmony in the development profile, attachment and dissociation. This information is provided in this chapter.

## 4.1 What is trauma?

The word trauma has been heard with increasing frequency in the last few years and is now so often used in so many contexts that there is a danger of losing sight of the actual definition of the word. The word trauma is often used to refer to a shocking, negative event and also to the consequences which this event has or could have on a person's life. This is actually untrue; the word 'trauma' points only to the event itself and not to people's reactions. This term should only be used for serious negative events which have been, or could be, overwhelming in a psychological way for those involved.

### 4.1.1 Trauma and DSM

In this book we aim to correlate information to the DSM-5 (*Diagnostic and Statistical Manual of Mental Disorders*, fifth edition) as much as possible. The source of information about the DSM-5 is the website www.dsm5.org.

The DSM-5 describes a trauma as a psychological reaction to exposure to a direct threat or a personal experience in which a person is confronted with serious injuries, death or sexual violence. Sexual violence is explicitly mentioned here (in contrast with the earlier DSM-IV).

Exposure is connected to one of the following scenarios, in which the individual:

- experiences the traumatic event themselves
- witnesses the event personally
- finds out that a close family member or friend has experienced a traumatic event (which concerns the threat of death caused by violence or an accident)
- is repeatedly personally subject to extreme aversive details of a traumatic event.[1]

The reaction to this event is so serious that it has a clinically significant and/or invalidating effect on the social interactions of the person involved, their ability to work and other important areas of functioning. It must be excluded that these effects are caused by medical conditions, medication, drugs or alcohol.

Four diagnostic clusters are defined which describe the behaviour, these being:

1. *Intrusions:* spontaneous memories of the traumatic event which describe the behaviour, repetitive dreams related to what has happened, flashbacks and intense, continuous psychological disruption.
2. *Avoidance behaviour:* avoiding internally disruptive memories, thoughts or feelings and avoiding external situations which remind the person of the event.
3. *Negative cognitions and moods:* varying from persistent disturbed cognitions in which, for example, unjustified feelings of guilt and accusations play a role, a strange feeling with regard to other people, less interest in activities, to memory problems with regard to what has happened.
4. *Irritability:* in which reckless, aggressive or self-destructive behaviour, sleeping problems,hyper alertness and associated problems play a role.

Contrary to the old DSM-IV, the DSM-5 also pays attention to the 'fight reactions' to trauma, alongside attention to the co-called 'flight reactions' (see also Section 4.2.2).

The DSM-5 also includes a sub-type in which post-traumatic stress reactions in children younger than six years are described. In children, disorganised and agitated behaviour is generally seen and it is less possible to define the independent diagnostic clusters.

Pathology is indicated only when stress symptoms occur for a long period of time, bringing considerable suffering alongside them.[2] In this case, one speaks of a post-traumatic stress disorder (PTSD).

Due to the fact that the exact criteria and classification of the symptoms were not available at the time of writing, we have chosen to also use the DSM-IV-TR. To clarify the difference between PTSD and an acute stress disorder we refer to the diagnostic criteria which can be found online.

In the DSM-IV, acute stress disorder is also described. This diagnosis is given when symptoms of PTSD, especially dissociative symptoms, occur within a month after the traumatic event has taken place.

### 4.1.2 Types of trauma

There are different types of trauma. First there is acute trauma. This is a single event which lasts for a short length of time.[3] Examples of this are a single incident of rape, being involved in a car crash, the death of a loved one, violence on the street or experiencing a robbery. This form of trauma is also called type I trauma.[4]

In type II trauma (or chronic trauma) there is long-term, repetitive violence, danger, threats or (sexual) abuse. Chronic trauma can also occur due to a build-up of various traumatic experiences, for example the death of a partner, experiencing a serious accident of a child and being the victim of a robbery.

A third form of trauma is complex trauma. Complex trauma describes a specific form of chronic trauma and the effect it has on victims. This consists of repeated traumatic events which generally begin at a very young age (before the age of five years). It is caused by adults who should be caring for and protecting the child. Typical of this form of trauma is that attachment problems (the adult should actually have been protecting and/or comforting and supporting the child after the trauma) go hand-in-hand with overwhelming negative experiences. An example of a complex trauma is continuing maltreatment and sexual abuse which start at a young age and are perpetrated by parents and/or other caregivers.[5]

Finally, it is often the case that people who have been confronted with others who have experienced a traumatic event develop stress symptoms themselves. These symptoms arise due to the impact of the stories of the victims and are referred to as secondary traumatising. Secondary trauma is described by Figley[6] as:

> the natural behaviour and emotions which follow finding out about a traumatic event which is experienced by a significant

> other... The stress which occurs due to helping or wanting to offer help to a traumatised or suffering person.

This concept can concern close relatives, but also healthcare professionals. The symptoms of secondary traumatic stress are similar to those of post-traumatic stress. Intrusions, avoidance and heightened irritability can be experienced as well as sleeping problems and loss of concentration.[7]

## 4.2 Trauma – what happens in the brain?

The consequences of trauma are far-reaching: many traumatised people face problems of a psychological and social nature. Until now the explanations for this were only sought in psychology. Neurobiology, however, shows (by use, among others things, of EEG and MRI) that sexual abuse and other forms of serious and long-term stress also have vast consequences for the structure, volume and function of the brain.[8]

The physical structure of the brain is dynamic. This means that the brain structure, with certain boundaries, comes into being in interaction with the environment. The number of receptors in the brain for certain neurotransmitters and hormones can increase or decrease as a reaction to stress. It is also known that the activity of neurotransmitters and hormones change, both in the brain as in the other parts of the body (such as the adrenal glands).

### 4.2.1 The structure of the brain

To be able to understand the issue of trauma, it is important to know how the brain is constructed and which parts of the brain play a role in the perception and experience of trauma.

These parts are interconnected, but each controls a separate series of functions. The brainstem regulates the most important physical regulatory functions, such as body temperature, heartbeat, breath and blood pressure. The midbrain and the limbic system regulate emotional reactions which control our behaviour. The top part of the brain (the cerebral cortex) regulates the complicated functions such as language and speech, abstract thought, plans and conscious decision making.[10]

**Table 4.1 The construction of the brain**[9]

| | |
|---|---|
| Cerebral cortex | Abstract thought<br>Concrete thought<br>Affiliation (connectedness) |
| Limbic system | 'Attachment'<br>Sexual behaviour<br>Emotional behaviour<br>Regulation of movement |
| Midbrain | 'Sensations'<br>Appetite/feeling full |
| Brainstem | Sleep<br>Blood pressure<br>Heart rhythm<br>Body temperature |

The brain develops according to a fixed and hierarchic order from the least complex (brainstem and midbrain) to the most complex (the cerebral cortex).[11] This is also referred to as the primitive and the more complex brain.[12] The primitive brain controls the basic functions and reactions which are necessary to survive. It enables us to make fast, reflex decisions which protect us in dangerous situations. The more complex brain is responsible for abstract thought, plans, reasoning and conscious processing of information.

### 4.2.2 The brain and stress

What happens when people experience bad things? If a person is in danger, a sort of alarm bell in the brain is activated which initiates the so-called 'fight-flight-freeze mechanism'.[13] This mechanism is an active defence against danger and can be compared with the strategies which animals use in order to survive: fight, flight or freeze.[14]

The fight-flight-freeze mechanism works under the influence of the stress hormones adrenaline and cortisol. Adrenaline is released within a few seconds and causes physiological reactions, such as raised heartbeat, quicker breathing, increased blood pressure, increased blood supply to the skeleton and heightened alertness.[15]

If a stressful situation lasts longer than 20 minutes then cortisol is released. Cortisol makes extra energy available and inhibits the stress reaction in order to prevent exhaustion.

Parts of the more complex segment of the brain then help in analysing the threat of danger. If the threat of danger is assessed as being 'not serious' then the primitive brain receives a sign to stop producing the stress hormone so the body can function normally again.[16]

In most cases, the body's reaction to the emergency situation stops shortly after the danger has passed. In the case of chronic traumatising, this system remains active and the primitive brain keeps producing stress hormones. The body has no chance of recovering. The continuous production of stress hormones possibly explains the frequent occurrence of infections in seriously traumatised people.[17]

Cortisol takes over the function of the immune system for a while; in long-term stress this immune system becomes lazy. In addition, the influence of cortisol makes people constantly alert in order to be able to survive in a threatening environment. If the primitive brain continues to produce stress hormones this makes it more difficult for the more complex segment of the brain, which applies functions such as thinking and planning, to function efficiently.[18] Many people who experience a chronic trauma demonstrate disorders such as a lack of concentration and hyper-alert behaviour. This trauma-related behaviour is often confused with attention deficit hyperactivity disorder (ADHD), especially when seen in children.

### 4.2.3 The influence of trauma on the brain structure

An area which has received an increasing amount of attention in the past decades is the research into the effects of maltreatment and neglect on the development of the brain during early childhood. Based on this research, it is now stated that trauma has an effect on the structure of the brain. This provides biological explanations for that which therapists of traumatised clients had previously described in physiological and emotional terms and in terms of behaviour.[19]

In seriously emotionally neglected children, in comparison with children who were not abused, a smaller brain size and a decrease in the cerebral cortex is observed.[20] There are also indications that the cerebral cortex is less thick in victims of long-term abuse.[21]

A basic division could be made in the functions of the right and left half of the brain: left for neutral memories, logical thought and language-focused functions and right for visual-spatial functions and coping with (negative) emotions. In literature on the subject, the verbal IQ is traditionally connected to the left half of the brain and the perceptual reasoning IQ to the right half of the brain.[22]

In traumatised children, the left half of the brain is generally less developed. The brain areas which are responsible for the activity state of the brain, coping with emotions, memory and learning are affected by chronic traumatising.[23]

Traumatised children can react in strong emotional ways and are less able to regulate their emotions with cognitions. This possibly clarifies the very large discrepancy between verbal IQ and perceptual reasoning IQ in many children who have experienced sexual abuse.

## 4.3 Reactions to trauma

Everybody reacts differently to traumatic events. Their reaction depends on various factors, such as age, developmental phase and temperament. A trauma at a young age can have long-lasting effects, sometimes far into adulthood. This is due to the fact that the personalities of young people are still strongly in development and experiencing a trauma can negatively influence this development.[24] Also of importance is whether or not the victim has understood the danger and how the danger is perceived. Alongside the age and the developmental phase, temperament is a decisive factor for the way in which a person reacts to a shocking event. Some people have a more anxious and sensitive nature, while others are more resilient and not so easily upset.

The reaction to trauma is also influenced by possible other traumatic experiences. The more trauma present in the life history of a person, the more difficult it is to cope with a new event.[25]

Finally, the way in which people in the surrounding social environment react to the traumatic event and the presence of emotional and social support are of great influence to the reaction to stress. This is especially the case in people with an intellectual disability due to the greater dependency on others around them.

### 4.3.1 Coping process

Coping with a traumatic experience is a process in which stress reactions generally occur.

Stress reactions can be divided into four categories:

- intrusion
- avoidance or disengagement
- heightened irritability
- negative cognition and moods.

*Intrusion* means that people relive the traumatic event with repetitive and drastically unpleasant memories of it. These images and memories arise during quiet situations or when the person is alone. People can, both physically and emotionally, react in severe ways to things which remind them of the traumatic event. These can include sounds, scents, tastes, places and people; these are called trauma-reminders (or triggers). The content and the form of the intrusion depend on the development of the memory and the ability to integrate the various senses in a memory. Nightmares can occur about the traumatic event. Traumatised children often suffer from frightening dreams without recognisable content. Another specific intrusion reaction in children is post-traumatic play.[26]

In *avoidance or disengagement,* people try to avoid all memories of the traumatic event. They don't want to talk about it, they avoid places, things or people which remind them of the event, or they deny that it happened. Avoidance can occur consciously, but also unconsciously.

*Heightened irritability* is demonstrated by exaggerated watchfulness and being startled, as if the person is constantly aware of new danger. People are exaggeratedly alert and aware (hyper-vigilance) and easily startled. These people can have difficulty concentrating, find it difficult to go to sleep or to sleep through the night and can become angry or fearful quickly.

*Negative cognition and moods.* Seriously disturbed cognitions can occur, in which, for example, unjustified guilt or accusations can play a role. People can also lose pleasure in certain activities and hobbies and have the feeling of being numb or separated from normal life. This flatness of emotions can create a feeling of alienation and loneliness, with negative thoughts about the future.

It is important to emphasise that the reactions described are normal reactions to extreme events and will generally lessen within a number of weeks, and eventually disappear.

### 4.3.2 Dissociation

A specific reaction to trauma is dissociation. Dissociation can best be described as a narrowed consciousness.[27] Emotional events do not penetrate to the 'personal' consciousness. Emotional retreat is a way to deal with the overwhelming stress of the traumatic event. In full dissociation the person appears to 'be absent for a while', the images of the event are separated from the daily consciousness. When the person 'returns again' he often does not know what has happened.

In partial dissociation people do experience the traumatic event but do not feel emotions or physical sensations; the person looks at him/herself from a distance. These people can talk about the event afterwards, but there is a memory loss about the traumatic feelings and sensations. These people can often talk about the shocking event in a (too) sober way, which should not be confused with coping with the event well.[28]

Young children develop the tendencies for dissociation more easily than older children and adults. In the case of chronic traumatising it appears that the sooner in life the traumatic events start, the larger the chance that tendencies for dissociation will develop.[29] According to Professor Frank Putnam – connected to the Mayerson Center for Safe and Healthy Children and UC Department of Paediatrics and one of the world's most important researchers in the field of trauma and dissociation in children and adolescents – these tendencies concern a developmental phenomenon with a peak at the age of ten, which subsequently decreases during adolescence and adulthood.[30] For specific information about dissociation in people with an intellectual disability see Section 4.6.3.

### 4.3.3 Other associated disorders

A trauma can also lead to other psychiatric disorders, other than an acute stress disorder, dissociation, which can occur alongside PTSD. An overview by Deering and colleagues shows that PTSD seldom occurs alone.[31] Comorbidity of PTSD with fear and depression is especially high.[32] It is possible that these psychiatric disorders were present before the traumatic event. In that case, these disorders can increase the vulnerability towards experiencing drastic events and the inadequate ability to cope with them.

Finally, it should be noted that not everyone who experiences a serious trauma develops PTSD.[33] Good support after experiencing a traumatic event and a supportive and understanding reaction from significant others is essential. The SOS handbook provides a valuable contribution to organising this support.

## 4.4 Age-specific reactions to traumatic events

The stress reactions of avoidance, heightened irritability and intrusion occur in different amounts in most adults who experience a shocking event. The PTSD concept, as described in the DSM, is based on experiences with adults without an intellectual disability and insufficiently describes the occurrence and reactions in children, adolescents and people with a disability, especially in the case of type II trauma.[34] Many children and adolescents react to a single traumatic experience with behaviour described in the DSM-IV as traumatic play, (frightening) dreams, restlessness and avoidance behaviour. But mainly general symptoms and complaints occur which are connected to the developmental age of the child, such as psychosomatic complaints, toilet training problems, concentration problems, attention-seeking behaviour, retreat, resistance and anger.[35]

In people, with or without a disability, who have experienced very negative events for a long period of time (such as sexual abuse and neglect), the PTSD concept is then even more insufficient than in the case of single traumas. Putnam[36] says: 'It should be recognised that most traumatised children do not officially qualify as having PTSD. For traumatised children there are deeper wounds beyond PTSD.'

Children demonstrate different reactions, depending on various factors, including the age and the developmental phase. The next sections provide descriptions of the stress reactions which are specific to the various age phases (see also Table 4.2).

### 4.4.1 Reactions in babies to traumatic events

Babies are completely dependent on their parents. Babies check the facial expressions of the parents to determine whether a situation is safe or not. This is called 'social referencing'. Babies also need their parents to reassure them. If parents themselves have been exposed to traumatic situations they are often not in a state to reassure the baby. The stress reaction of the parent is then also a risk factor for the baby in developing trauma complaints.

Babies often express trauma-related complaints through sleeping and eating problems and frequent and long-lasting crying.[37] In addition, there is a heightened risk of a disturbance in the development of the attachment between the parents and the baby. Due to the fact that the parent is not in an adequate state to calm their child, anxious attachment behaviour occurs. The stress system of the baby does not calm down and remains 'alert'.

### 4.4.2 Reactions in toddlers and young children to traumatic events

Toddlers and young children have many important developmental tasks. In interpreting external threats, these young children mainly rely on the reaction of their parents and are above all dependant on the coping skills of their parents. In traumatic events, a disturbance can occur between the attachment between parent and child.

Toddlers and young children especially suffer from fear of separation as a reaction to trauma. They can be extremely scared of strangers. Young children often cope with the themes of the shocking event in repetitive solo play. Repeating the same type of play, with no development in the play, is often seen in such situations. Sleepwalking, talking in their sleep, nightmares, general restlessness and irritability, poor listening skills, watchfulness and being startled quickly also occur at this age.

Young children aged four to six cannot yet see the perspective of the other person and have not yet mastered the thought process of cause and effect. This developmental phase that is characterised by magical thinking can lead to self-blame and confusion, which can be translated in behavioural terms to an increase in temper tantrums, worrying or 'clamping behaviour'. Clamping behaviour originates from the fear of letting the carer go, in case something bad happens to them or the child.[38, 39, 40] Young children also often react with regressive behaviour, especially in the area of language and toilet training. In addition there can also be a delay in achieving the developmental milestones.

### 4.4.3 Reactions in school children to traumatic events

School children live more independent lives and are increasingly able to look after themselves. From about the age of six, children can put themselves in the position of another person, which can make them worry about others a lot. Children of this age often hesitate to bother their parents with bad experiences or complaints. They also have a lively imagination. They need to look for explanations of what has happened. They lack the ability to understand the actual facts and then fantasise about a cause and often seek this in themselves, with feelings of guilt arising as a result.

The following symptoms are specific in school children: trauma-related fears, physical complaints, sleeping problems, concentration problems, intrusive thoughts or nightmares, disturbed perception of time during the event, a changed attitude towards people, life and the future and thinking that there were omens by which they could have determined what was about to happen (the so-called 'omen-formation').[41, 42, 43, 44]

Many of the above mentioned reactions are expressed by school children in their play or in drawings. Instead of solo-play, which is seen in toddlers and young children, these children involve their friends in post-traumatic play. Re-enactment and re-victimising can occur in these situations. Re-enactment literally means: 'being performed again'. Children play out what has happened to them, but this time no longer as victim but as director in the game. The situation which the child passively experienced is actively expressed in their behaviour. Characteristic of re-enactment is that the person does not actually realise that they are repeating the traumatic experience. These are usually drastic and repeated experiences, which the person does not want to think about.[45] In the case of sexual abuse, children can demonstrate sexually inappropriate behaviour towards other children. To prevent the child feeling rejected, it is important to see these behavioural problems in relation to the traumatic event.

In re-victimisation, the child manoeuvres themselves unintentionally into a situation, in which a repeat of the experienced event occurs and the child is once again made the victim.

### 4.4.4 Reactions in teenagers and adolescents to traumatic events

Reactions in teenagers and adolescents are increasingly similar to those of adults. PTSD complaints can occur, but also other anxiety complaints, such as a general anxiety disorder or phobia. Teenagers and adolescents find it difficult to talk about their feelings regarding the trauma. This can increase the chance of developing feelings of depression; this is expressed in not being interested in doing things any more, no desire for contact with others, little appetite and limited future perspective.[46]

Suppressed feelings can also be expressed by young people as difficult and aggressive behaviour, resulting in conflicts with those around them. Auto-mutilation, risky and thrill-seeking behaviour and alcohol and drug use can become forms of self-medication in this age group as a reaction to traumatic events. In practice, this behaviour is often considered part of puberty, without seeing the meaning of the behaviour in light of the trauma. The consequence is that treatment in young people is often aimed at changes in behaviour, with no attention paid to the underlying trauma.

Central in the developmental phase of young people (Table 4.1) is the development of autonomy, where orientation towards friends increases. This development is related in a difficult way to the feeling of vulnerability and being overwhelmed by a traumatic experience. A role as victim, and having to accept help, is at odds with the desire to be independent and self-reliant. In the case of sexual abuse it is sometimes seen that young people claim to have chosen the relationship with (and/or to be in love with) the perpetrator of the abuse. Only in this way can the autonomy be kept intact. Finally, due to their capability for abstract reasoning, teenagers and adolescents are able to think about how a certain situation could have been avoided. Negative cognitions arise about themselves in which young people judge themselves, and these can lead to developing a strong feeling of guilt.[47]

**Table 4.2 Behavioural signals (sexual) abuse**

| Babies and toddlers | Infants | School children (5–12 years) | Early adolescence (12–14 years) | Late adolescence (15–18 years) |
|---|---|---|---|---|
| Poor development | Aggressive behaviour | Intimidating behaviour | Violence in relations with others | Violence in relations with others |
| Apathy | Dependence | General aggression | Intimidating behaviour | Excessive alcohol and drug use |
| Disturbance in eating and sleeping habits | Fear | Depression | Low self-worth | Running away from home |
| Developmental disorders | Cruelty towards animals | Fear | Suicide | Sudden drop in presence at school and school achievement |
| | Vandalism of possessions | Lack of respect for women; stereotypical ideas about male-female roles | Lack of respect for women; stereotypical ideas about male-female roles | Lack of respect for women; stereotypical ideas about male-female roles |

*cont.*

| **Babies and toddlers** | **Infants** | **School children (5–12 years)** | **Early adolescence (12–14 years)** | **Late adolescence (15–18 years)** |
|---|---|---|---|---|
| | Symptoms of PTSD | Symptoms of PTSD | Truanting from school | |
| | | Unruly behaviour | Worrying about their own body | |
| | | Vandalism of possessions | Symptoms of PTSD | |
| | | Poor school results | | |
| | | Disengagement | | |

## 4.5 Coping with trauma

Recovery after a traumatic event is generally referred to as 'coping'. Coping with a traumatic experience is a process in which stress reactions occur. These normal stress reactions largely overlap with PTSD symptoms: intrusions, avoidance and increased irritability. These are normal reactions to extreme events!

Traumatic experiences disturb the peace, safety and certainty of everyday life. The normality of daily life and the trust in other people is roughly disturbed. Coping with this shock means building or recovering a sense of balance, so that people can live without being constantly confronted by thoughts and feelings about the traumatic event and the associated images. It is a process in which re-finding a sense of control in one's own existence takes a central place.

Coping with a traumatic event does not mean that the person has no more problems or sadness. The traumatic event remains a part of the life and history of the person. Coping with a traumatic event means that a person succeeds in achieving a new sense of balance and therefore can integrate the traumatic event (including the consequences) into their life – alongside all the good and bad things that have happened.

Safety is an important concept in being able to cope with a traumatic event. A person must be safe in order to cope; this means that the real danger no longer exists (for example, in the case of sexual abuse, the abuse must have stopped). Safety also means a feeling of safety; this perception of safety is often separate from physical safety. The development of a feeling of safety depends on the emotions and social support which a person receives after experiencing a traumatic event. In addition, age, developmental phase and general temperament are influential factors in the way in which a person copes with a traumatic event (see Section 4.3).

### 4.5.1 Psychological rumination

Alongside elements which can be beneficial to the coping with trauma, there are also issues which can stand in the way of the process. People often say (well meaningly) after a shocking event: 'You mustn't think about it too much. Try to forget about it', or, 'You must look towards the future. Why don't you stop thinking about it? There are so many other beautiful things in the world.'

In the first place, it is difficult to follow this advice. How can someone do this? The thoughts about the shocking event automatically arise! It is actually not good advice. At the best of times this will only provide a little relief. It means that the 'process of psychological rumination' cannot occur. Feelings and thoughts which are connected to the traumatic event do not have the chance of diminishing. People are then continuously trying to avoid images, sounds and events which remind them of the trauma. A confrontation with these factors causes the feelings and memories to arise in full severity. People run the risk of finding themselves in a vicious circle. However, during the process of 'psychological rumination' the overwhelming traumatic event is, as it were, divided into small pieces of information. In this way, the information can gradually be given a place in the wholeness of experiences.[48] Time heals many wounds in coping with trauma. As previously discussed, stress reactions are considered as a disorder only when the complaints last for a longer period and cause considerable suffering (see Section 4.1.1).

## 4.6 Trauma and coping with trauma in people with an intellectual disability

People have long thought that those with an intellectual disability, like young children, would not be troubled by psychological problems and trauma-related issues. Fortunately, this school of thought has ceased to exist in the last 20 years. There is no argument needed anymore to conclude that they, just as any other person, do actually suffer from problems related to trauma. People with an intellectual disability experience the consequences of shocking events, such as sexual abuse.[49, 50] The impact on the life of the person is generally such that there are far-reaching consequences for the quality of life. The complaints often manifest themselves via behavioural problems and the trauma component in the diagnostics is therefore not considered. There is a danger of the treatment focusing on preventing the behavioural problems and of the underlying issues not being treated.

Research by Sequera and Hollins demonstrates that the same trauma symptoms occur in people with an intellectual disability as in those without an intellectual disability.[51] The symptoms and anxieties are, however, linked to their mental age and correspond less with the calendar age. Not only is cognitive functioning linked to the mental age, but also the social and emotional level of functioning.[52] People with a severe intellectual disability suffer sensory overstimulation more frequently, which can result in powerful reactions to loud sounds and the dark. The symptoms are expressed in their behaviour, for example by inconsolable crying, screaming, aggression or destructive and/or self-injuring behaviour (see Section 4.4.1). Symptoms such as these are also seen in people with a mild or moderate intellectual disability and a lower level of social and emotional development. In people with a mild or moderate intellectual disability, depending on the (developmental) age, post-traumatic symptoms are often expressed via behaviour, such as introverted regressive behaviour, inhibition of movement, over-sexualised behaviour, thrill-seeking behaviour and alcohol or drug abuse.

### *Syndromes*

It is important to realise that people with an intellectual disability often have an additional syndrome. It is known that anxiety plays a role in various syndromes. The DSM (the DM-ID, Diagnostic Manual for Intellectual Disabilities)[53] includes a chapter about a number of syndromes. From research into behavioural phenotypes, a link is made to psychiatric symptoms and disorders. Syndromes which can be named here are: Down syndrome, FAS (foetal alcohol syndrome), Fragile-X syndrome, PKY (phenylketonuria), Prader-Willi syndrome, Smith-Magenis syndrome, Velo-cardio-facial syndrome (VCF) and Williams syndrome. People with these syndromes have a high level of vulnerability towards developing serious anxiety and compulsive behaviour as a reaction to stressful circumstances. In clients with FAS, a past history without attachment problems, neglect and violence is almost unthinkable due to the cause of the syndrome. Seeing this behaviour as purely arising from and being part of the syndrome, without considering the possibility of a trauma reaction, does not lead to adequate treatment of the underlying problems.

### *Limited integrative ability*

It is clear that people with an intellectual disability suffer from psychological disorders more often than those without a disability. The cause of this lies in the heightened psychological vulnerability which is connected to a limited integrative ability, in comparison to people without a disability.[54] It is more difficult for people with an intellectual disability to cope with stress. This is due to the fact that, partly because of their lower cognitive level, they have less complex and active coping mechanisms available to deal with the problems and stresses of life. Complex coping mechanisms are connected to metacognitive abilities (flexible and abstract thought), which people with an intellectual disability generally do not fully possess. This applies to 'normal' stress which people experience in everyday life, but of course even more so in coping with the stress caused by a traumatic experience. It is therefore not surprising that there are indications that people with an intellectual disability have a greater chance of developing PTSD symptoms.[55]

### 4.6.1 Coping with trauma and a disharmonic developmental profile

In people with an intellectual disability there is also often a difference between the intellectual ability and social and emotional functioning: a so-called disharmonic developmental profile. The social and emotional development remains far behind cognitive development. This discrepancy leads to the way in which people with an intellectual disability are often overrated in their emotional resilience. On the basis of the cognitive (most visible) functioning, people appear to be able to do more than they actually can cope with emotionally. This low capability level can lead to symptoms which are related to a lower emotional developmental phase than people would expect on the grounds of the calendar age and cognitive development.

An interesting question, which is extremely relevant here, is how do these differences in the developmental areas arise? This calls for a closer consideration of the process of development regarding people with an intellectual disability in general. The personality development of people with a disability is a fragile development. They are influenced by a complex combination of personal factors and environmental influences. This vulnerable development leads to a raised prevalence of behavioural problems and emotional and relationship problems.[56] Everyone is born with the natural tendency to integrate experiences in a coherent life history, and with a realisation of who they are. Our integrative ability makes us able to distinguish the past and the present and to stay aware in the present when we think about the past or about our future. This ability also helps us to develop self-awareness.

The safer the emotional and physical environment in which we grow up, the better we are able to continue to develop and strengthen this integrative ability. In the course of this development, we connect our life experiences and how we interact and in this way we form our sense of self.[57]

For people with an intellectual disability, there are many issues starting from a young age when it comes to the social and emotional development and the sense of self. They learn from a young age that they do not fit into the group and cannot keep up with others. They unconsciously feel the disappointment of their parents of not being that which the parents had hoped for.[58] They experience the way in which younger brothers and sisters or children living near them pass them by and the way in which they themselves cannot keep up at school. They also experience in all sorts of situations that they are slower than others and that their reactions are different. Bullying is also often reported.

At a later age, implicit social rejection can be experienced, that of living in a world which does everything to prevent people such as themselves from being born.[59] Additionally, multiple studies conclude that sexual abuse, maltreatment and neglect, also at a young age, occur much more frequently in those with an intellectual disability than those without an intellectual disability.[60]

Furthermore, for many of the clients for whom the SOS handbook is written, an out-of-home placement(s) and the loss of the trusted environment play a role. In the case of people who have been placed in a care home group, the loss of trusted others who look after you naturally and the lack of personal involvement are also significant. Van IJzendoorn and colleagues speak of 'structural neglect'[61] due to the unavoidable discontinuity in care and the unavoidable unreliability in the upbringing/professional care work. It is also the case that people live in a care home group in which, as a result of the issues of those around them, violence or threats of violence are part of their daily reality. Sometimes the client is the victim, sometimes they witnesses violence or sense the continuous hyper-alertness of those who are meant to protect them. It is unavoidable that this build-up of strong negative emotions will have an effect on people. The above mentioned issues could be considered as being 'potentially traumatic events'. It is a natural course of events that the social and emotional development will stagnate further considering the predisposition for avoidant coping behaviour which arises from these complex circumstances.

Valarie Sinason, the English psychoanalyst with much experience in treating people with an intellectual disability who have been sexually abused, speaks in this context of the 'handicapped smile'. She maintains that what is often seen as an expression of naive content in characterising people with an intellectual disability ('They're such happy people…') can also be seen as a significant diagnostic sign of pain and suffering. This corresponds to the concept of Selma Freiberg, who speaks of 'affect transformation'. This means that children who find themselves in long-lasting traumatic circumstances, from which they cannot escape due to their dependency, give in and adapt by continually grinning and/or fully or partially starting to function on a lower level.[62]

In Dutch-speaking countries, age equivalents are often used for the various developmental areas in order to make the social environment aware of the discrepancy in development and to avoid over-expectations. It is questionable whether the concept of a disharmonic developmental profile, with the related age equivalents, actually does justice to the origin of the issues. Considering the developmental process we have described here, it may be better to speak of clients with an untreated chronic and complex trauma, with, as a consequence, disintegration between the various developmental areas. Treatment is required and should be aimed at coping with chronic trauma in general, with the focus on integration and balance between the various developmental areas.

### 4.6.2 Attachment and coping with trauma

The basis of the development of a child is made in the attachment relationship, which begins to develop at birth. This starts from the moment that a relationship forms around the regulation of arousal, sleeping and waking, hunger and feeling full, and lust and aversion. For people with an intellectual disability, this relationship is under pressure from the start.[63] This pressure is due to the increased vulnerability of the parents who may be worried and have the idea that there is something unusual about their newborn child, or who are coming to terms with the fact that their child has a disability. These are factors which complicate the necessary susceptibility and availability of the parent towards the emotional needs of this special child.

There are also 'damaging circumstances' on the child's side. The child may send out weaker signs, making it difficult for the parents to understand what the child needs and for them to respond effectively. The child can also (if they have had a lot of pain and experienced suffering) experience the world as being frightening and painful instead of safe and caring, despite all the good support that the parents provide. In these situations, the parents miss the positive experience of 'understanding' their child, getting to know the child and being able to comfort them, and subsequently the child cannot be comforted. This results in the parents lacking the fundaments for feeling competent about their parenting, and the child experiencing the world as an unsafe place. A safe attachment is a good start for the continuation of the development of personality. A child who is safely attached can be compared to a house with a firm foundation. All sorts of things can happen in the further building which decide the definitive adult house, but the chance of a strong house is greater if there is a firm foundation.

Various research points to the way in which safely attached children function better in all domains of life. With regard to the social development, children who are safely attached can easily seek for help from adults and are able to interact with them better. They are also more communicative, because they have experienced that others are there to listen to them and to help them when needed. Above all, social development and the development of the sense of self are strongly related. A child who feels loved builds a sense of self, of being someone who is worthwhile. In comparison, a child who never feels understood starts thinking of themselves as 'strange or bad' and not being worthwhile to listen to.

Ricky Greenwald, clinical psychologist and founder of the Child Trauma Institute in the US, states that attachment is also strongly related to coping style.[64] If the child has experienced a mother who is 'good enough', then the child will have learnt that bad experiences (hunger, thirst, being angry, pain), even though they are not pleasant experiences, are actually things that they can cope with and that everything will eventually be all right again. If these children are confronted by memories of traumatic situations, they will have adopted the experience and coping style in order to withstand difficult circumstances. Children with problematic attachment styles have learnt from experience that if they feel rough, they cannot depend on another person to help them. They know that these feelings can be overwhelming and disastrous. They learn that bad feelings can be dangerous and that they should be avoided as much as possible. In a trauma situation, these children display a tendency towards avoidance and dissociation.

### 4.6.3 Dissociation and people with an intellectual disability

Dissociation starts when an experience is so threatening and overwhelming at a certain moment that the client is not able to (fully) integrate the experience into their sense of self and life story. It is a primitive avoidance coping reaction, which is also often seen in young children in threatening circumstances, in which the brain is fully or partially cut off or split as a survival strategy in overwhelming experiences. Lessened consciousness occurs. The client is, as it were, 'absent' for a while. The images of the experience are disconnected from daily consciousness at the moment that the experience becomes too powerful to regulate or comprehend in another way. When the client 'comes back' and 'is there again', they do not know, or hardly know what has happened; they suffer full or partial memory loss about the event. In this way clients can experience the most terrible things and despite this appear to be carrying on with daily life. It seems as if nothing is wrong and that they are not bothered by anything (see also Section 4.1.1).

Alongside a higher vulnerability towards developing PTSD symptoms, people with an intellectual disability also more often suffer dissociative complaints. Biological, social and environmental factors influence the vulnerability towards dissociation. People with an intellectual disability are less able to integrate traumatic experiences than those without an intellectual disability, due to the way in which the brain is developed. At a neurological and biological level, certain development of the brain and of the neural network is required for the integration to go well. The sense of self and the personality development often show less coherence as they are already under pressure (also see the other paragraphs in Section 4.6). This increases the risk of dissociation, especially when people are not able to rely on sufficient social and emotional support and if there is a history of abuse, maltreatment and neglect.[65]

Much research[66] has shown that such histories occur more frequently in people with an intellectual disability than in those without an intellectual disability (see also Section 4.6.1). A risk factor also lies here with regard to social and emotional support. Adults and children with an intellectual disability, particularly when they have been taken into a care home group and stay in the institution, generally have a very limited network and scarce support from professionals in their upbringing, as these professionals also have many other clients to look after.

### Dissociation and intrusions

Dissociation during trauma is unfortunately ineffective in the long term because the dissociated experiences often come back at unpredictable moments, for example in the form of intrusions. An intrusion means re-experiencing an event. The client experiences the traumatising event as if it was happening again.

An intrusion is triggered by something which reminds the client about the traumatising event. The client once again finds themselves in an overwhelming experience, which is just as powerful as the actual event, while in reality there is no danger. The intrusion can be so lifelike that it takes the client back in time. The perception of the client can be so disturbed that the face of the caregiver turns into the face of the perpetrator for the client at that moment. This is very frightening and can cause powerful reactions.

The trigger which causes the intrusion can be anything. Sometimes it is an actual thing which can be recognised by the people around the client, if they are aware of the trauma (such as a certain place or the colour of a car). It can also be a scent or an atmosphere, or the tone of voice, which makes the intrusion come as a complete surprise (often also for the client themselves). In this case, the client's powerful outbursts and behavioural problems seem to arise 'out of nowhere'.

Often caregivers assume that clients who dissociate in a milder form are not troubled by what they have experienced. Shortly after the abuse, still no alarming behaviour is seen; support and treatment do not seem to be necessary. If symptoms do develop in the long term, the link is often no longer made.

### Structural dissociation

If a client has an intrusion and cannot cope with the stress which this causes, dissociation occurs again. Once the brain has got used to dissociation, this then continues to be the preferred strategy (sometimes for years afterwards). This means that the client does not learn how they could deal with tension in another way and the brain uses this strategy sooner and more often. Eventually the client will start dissociating about things which are unimportant in the eyes of those around them.[67]

This circle can continue to strengthen itself and eventually disturb the integrative functions. This results in structural dissociation, in which the personality and consciousness are divided into different parts, which are in contact with each other and work together to varying degrees.[68] Clients generally describe such experiences as 'hearing voices'. The voices which are heard are related to the traumatic experience.[69]

It is also reported that there are 'pieces' in a person's head. Sinason[70] describes a client who expressed this aptly by saying, 'My poor brain broke into pieces!' The trouble is that professionals in the field still have little knowledge and awareness of this issue.[71] In the care of people with an intellectual disability, the disturbed integrative functions of clients with a trauma history are often wrongly viewed as being psychotic.[72]

In differential diagnostic terms, it is especially important to consider the type of the disintegration. If the disintegration and anxieties are related to the trauma, and the voices and parts which are reported can be seen as coming mainly from within the person's head, further investigations are strongly recommended. In these cases, an intensive trauma treatment, aimed at integration, should be considered before a treatment with antipsychotics.[73]

## SUMMARY

Various types of trauma can occur after a shocking event. Trauma affects the brain: stress hormones influence the structure of the brain and the way in which it works. General stress reactions are observed after experiencing a traumatic event, such as intrusions, heightened irritability and avoidance. If these stress reactions last for a long while and cause considerable suffering, this is referred to as a post-traumatic stress disorder. Other psychiatric disorders such as anxiety and depression can occur alongside this post-traumatic stress disorder. Specific reactions can occur per age group, in which dissociation can be seen as a specific reaction to trauma. The person who has experienced the traumatic event may not only develop symptoms, but secondary traumatic stress symtoms can also occur.

In people with an intellectual disability the same trauma symptoms occur as in people without a disability. The symptoms and anxieties are connected to the mental age and correspond less with the calendar age. Dissociative symptoms are seen more often in people with an intellectual disability. The development of personality in people with an intellectual disability is influenced by a complex combination of personal factors and environmental factors. This personality development can be strongly influence by diverse threats and potentially traumatic events. Treatment is required and should be aimed at coping with chronic trauma in general.

It is important to know that an extra sensitivity exists for people with certain syndromes to develop serious anxiety symptoms and often also compulsion symptoms after stressful circumstances. Interpreting this behaviour as being part of the syndrome, without considering the possibility of a trauma, usually does not lead to adequate treatment of the underlying trauma problems.

Chapter 5

# PSYCHOLOGICAL FIRST AID FOR CLIENTS WITH INTELLECTUAL DISABILITIES AFTER SEXUAL ABUSE

## Introduction

The moment of disclosure of sexual abuse is almost never announced in advance. It is often an unexpected situation for everybody. Even after long-lasting suspicions and a minimal fact interview, the actual confirmation of the suspicion still comes as a shock. Sometimes it is even a shock to clients themselves. Clients have often been living with a secret for a long time and this secret is suddenly out in the open. Their world has been turned upside down and all of a sudden everybody around them is involved. All focus is on the client, and, for some, this can be an overwhelming experience. Furthermore, all those involved around the client are affected by the disclosure – and may react differently from normal.

Daily life routines have changed all of a sudden as a result of the disclosure. With that change, a fundamental feeling of security is also lost.[1] This is an important factor in the support of people with a disability who have experienced sexual abuse.

In this chapter, we describe the core aspects of psychological first aid for clients with an intellectual disability. Helping the client feel safe is the main priority. Depending on their life history, people with a disability may react in varying ways to sexual abuse. It is important that professional caregivers consider the significance of the many possible client reactions, when seen in the light of the abuse. It is also crucial that professional caregivers remain calm when difficult behaviour is displayed.

This chapter provides a description of first aid support sessions between the professional and the victim with an intellectual disability (see Section 5.2). Attention is also given to the alignment of the SOS programme with the internal protocols of an organisation and the police. Alongside a concrete description of the sessions with the client, the needs of the client in daily life are also discussed in detail. These sessions are particularly intended for the support of people with a moderate or mild intellectual disability. Support for people with a severe intellectual disability is described in Chapter 7.

## 5.1 Core aspects for initial support

Incidences of sexual abuse can be extremely diverse. It makes an enormous difference whether the client was abused for a long time by a family member or was sexually approached on a single occasion by someone whom he or she hardly knew. Other influential factors include how intrusive the sexual acts were and whether or not the sexual abuse occurred in a trusted place. However, one cannot say that the consequences of sexual abuse directly depend on the details of the abuse. It is important to consider not only the details of the abuse, but also the characteristics of the client and their background as contributing factors to the consequences of the abuse. Additionally, the influence of adequate support from those in the client's immediate surroundings is essential, especially with regard to people with an intellectual disability.

Seen from a developmental perspective, the basic development or the developmental level of a client is a protective or risk-increasing factor in terms of the consequences of sexual abuse. In the same line of thought, literature on the subject states that the younger a child is at the time of abuse or maltreatment, the greater the risk of severe consequences.

The development of the personality of people with a disability is almost always an extremely fragile development. The client's development does not only increase the risk of abuse, but also increases the risk of severe consequences. Due to their cognitive disability, people with a disability have fewer coping mechanisms in place for dealing with stressful events (see Section 4.4). Furthermore, there is a high risk that people with an intellectual disability will be confronted with sexual abuse more than once in their lives, and may therefore already have suffered previous damage when a new case of abuse occurs. It is therefore important to consider the personal history of the client; an accumulation of experiences greatly reduces resilience. A client may sometimes react to minimal sexual stress factors in an extreme way (in the eyes of those around them). This reaction could be triggered by previous incidents of abuse (not always known about by professional caregivers and relatives).

### 5.1.1 Creating safety

In the first phase after the disclosure of sexual abuse, the first priority is to ensure the safety of all those involved. In practical terms, this means that the (suspected) perpetrator and victim are not confronted by each other's presence. It is often thought that separating the suspected perpetrator and victim is done to prevent a re-occurrence of the behaviour. This is an important factor, but additionally, the presence of the perpetrator in the daily life of the victim – their glances, movements and other non-verbal and possible verbal behaviour – results in the victim being constantly reminded of what has happened. It is almost impossible for the victim to experience a feeling of safety in such a situation, nor will the stress response system calm down. The internal alarm system is constantly 'switched on' by the presence of the (suspected) perpetrator. This makes coping with the situation impossible. When considering separating these people and creating a safe environment, attention should also be paid to creating safety in school and workplace situations, free-time activities, transport, and also with the use of social media.

With an eye to creating safety, it is also of great importance that structure, regularity and predictability in daily life are continued or, where necessary, reinstated. This is easier said than done in a situation in which all those involved have been upset and absorbed by what has come to light. There is a tendency towards letting boundaries fade, while thinking 'they have already experienced so much'. Although this attitude is understandable, it is, however, counterproductive. The client needs to experience a feeling of safety, and have caregivers who show them how to achieve this, especially in a period of upheaval. If the client lives in a group home, this does not only apply to the client themselves, but also to the other group members.

Safety not only concerns physical safety; a client must also actually *feel* safe. Alongside the stability of daily routines, it is also important to frequently send out safety messages. A safety message is a phrase or a statement in which the safety of the situation is emphasised, for example 'It is safe here', 'I will make sure that everything is OK here', 'Nothing can happen here'.

### *Informing others*

Safety also means that significant others, at places where the client regularly is, are aware of the abuse, so that they too can care for the client and provide adequate support. Places to inform are, for example: school, daytime activities, work, free-time clubs and addresses where the client stays the night. Other people to inform are group members, friends and relatives of the client.

It is possible that clients, in their upheaval, would prefer not to have significant others told about the abuse. In this case, it is important to explain to the client that they are not guilty regarding the abuse and that it is necessary that people around them know about it so that they can help.

Certainly in the case of people with a lower developmental level, a factor to be considered is that they have reduced awareness of cause and effect and are not completely sure of their own role in the process of abuse. Perpetrators often act by making clients jointly responsible ('We've got a secret game together', or 'You want this as well, don't you?') or by giving them something in exchange for the acts which the client carries out: presents, money, phone credit. From this viewpoint, the client may not want others to be informed about the abuse. They do not want to get into trouble about it. Clients also often find it difficult to think about what they could say and how they could formulate things to others. It is essential to help clients deal with this and, if required, to offer to do this for, or with, them. Keynotes to help initiate such conversations are included in the SOS programme and in the help book for the client (see Chapters 6 and 7).

### 5.1.2 Coping with stress reactions from the client

Dealing with a traumatic experience is a process in which stress reactions occur. It is important to emphasise that these reactions concern normal stress reactions to extreme events. These reactions shall generally lessen after a number of weeks and eventually cease to occur. If this is not the case and/or if there is considerable suffering caused by the after-effects, then therapeutic support is indicated.

When sexual abuse comes to light, the reactions of clients can be extremely diverse. Stress reactions can be divided into three categories: avoidance or disengagement, increased irritability and intrusion (see Chapter 4).

#### *Avoidance or disengagement*

Some clients appear to carry on as normal and do not seem to be troubled by what has happened. This can lead to a stress reaction in which the client, by simply carrying on with their daily life, avoids having to actually feel what has happened. These clients do not talk about what they have experienced and do not appear to be suffering.

It is, however, often reported that in such cases there are sudden unexpected behavioural changes or emotional outbursts. In many cases this concerns a trauma reaction to a trigger, which has not been recognised as such by the professional caregivers. In these situations, it is recommended that the caregivers initiate talking about the abuse in an easily approachable way, alongside the support sessions. In this way, experiences which have been hidden away can slowly 'land' in a safe way in daily life. It is important to communicate these initiatives as 'safety messages'. Safety messages are reassuring phrases in which caregivers express that the situation is safe, that the client is being looked after, that nothing can happen, that the abuse is no longer taking place.

#### *Increased irritability*

There are also clients who become extremely upset, cry a lot or display other intense reactions. In such situations it is important to explain to the client, and to those around them, that it is not unusual that people who have experienced something horrible are troubled by very strong feelings. These feelings can wash over you like waves and can make it difficult to pay attention to what is happening around you in the group, at school or at the day activity centre. It is logical that this happens, because the client's body again (or still) finds itself in a state of alarm at such moments. It is important, at such moments, that a client receives help from somebody who can help calm them down.

When a client is becoming extremely overwhelmed by their emotions, caregivers should not hesitate, but instead act straightaway in a proactive and active way. Clients can be helped to calm down in various ways. A general guideline is that the attention of the client should be directed outside themselves and towards making contact with the outside world. If the client is open for verbal communication, they can be made aware of the outside world by the caregiver simply saying things like, 'You are here in the group and everything is safe. Look around you, what can you see?' The client can be asked to describe what they can see in the room: 'What is in front of us? That is X's chair, what's next to it?' In this way, the client's attention is redirected from the internal and physical sensations and they should be able to come back into the present.[2]

It helps to let the client count from one to ten and, if that is too easy, count back from ten to one. It can also help to breathe deeply, together with the client, and make the out-breath last longer than the in-breath. This automatically signals the parasympathetic nervous system to relax. It is important to breathe together with the client and to act as an obvious role model. Behaving as a role model is essential, because clients subconsciously mirror the behaviour of significant others. Mirror neurons play an important part in this process.[3]

Clients are sometimes so disorientated that they can no longer be reached via language. The language system in the brain has been closed off as a consequence of the alarm phase.[4] At such moments, it is essential to find a way to reach them via the senses. This can be done by using a strong scent such as lavender or eucalyptus, or with strong chewing gum, for example. Another possibility is placing an ice cube in their hand. Movements (stamping, jumping, swinging and rocking) can also be used to help somebody make contact with the outside world. In this case, the professional caregivers also act as a role model.

It is important that the person offering the support remains calm themselves in all situations, with a 'calm brain'. Again, mirror neurons play a role here. Daniel Siegel, clinical psychiatrist, researcher and professor in neurobiology at the University of California, Los Angeles, elaborates on this context and talks about 'interpersonal neurobiology', in which he refers to the way that people subconsciously sense, copy and mutually regulate each other's biological state. In situations in which abuse has recently been disclosed, maintaining a calm brain is not a simple task for the professional caregivers (see Chapter 9).

### *Acting dependently*

The reaction of a client who has experienced sexual abuse largely depends on their past history. Clients who have had a troubled past and have experienced other relational traumas cannot fall back on a basic feeling of safety, due to the fact that this very experience is damaged. They don't have a stable image of safe relationships or the trust (or experience) that others are there to help them make the many unbearable emotions bearable. In their fear of having to cope alone, some clients act in an increasingly dependent way and make a heightened appeal on the emotional availability of the professional caregiver. These people clamp on to others out of fear, and sometimes also display anger and sadness the moment that the caregiver is not present.[5]

In such situations it is important to recognise the client's primitive need for attachment and to respond to this in a healthy way. If, however, this behaviour continues, this is an indication for seeking therapeutic help concerning attachment and trust. Experience teaches that such behaviour gradually lessens during a successful therapeutic process and is replaced by behaviour which is more appropriate to the (developmental) age.

### *Closing off from others*

There are also clients who turn away from trusted adults and prefer to go their own way. They often direct themselves indiscriminately towards other adults, with an eye towards meeting their basic needs, providing that the other adults fulfil their wishes. This is also considered an indication for therapeutic help.

#### *Intrusion*

Alongside the various reactions, there are also symptoms which are often suffered after sexual abuse. People who have been sexually abused often display sleeping problems. There are various reasons for this. First, many people are afraid of the dark. There is a natural disposition for people to feel more vulnerable when it is dark. Second, sleeping is an emotionally charged issue for many of those who have experienced sexual abuse, due to the fact that abuse often takes place in the evening or at night – and possibly in the same room in which the client is still sleeping. Finally, victims often have intrusions in their sleep or in the phase in between waking and sleeping, in the form of flashbacks or nightmares. In order to deal with these problems, it is important to explore with the client the ways in which the feeling of safety can be increased in the night. The client (and the people who are responsible for the night attendance) needs to be aware of the ways in which they can ask for help from the professional caregivers. It often helps to change the situation in the bedroom and, for example, to choose a different type of nightclothes from those the victim wore during the abuse. It can also help to purchase a night light or an extra listening system or baby monitor. In all cases, it is of great importance to introduce a fixed sleeping ritual to help the client acquire healthy habits in this area. In the worksheets (see Chapters 6 and 7) attention is given to a 'safe sleeping plan'.

### 5.1.3 Psychological first aid for other clients

When a victim of sexual abuse lives in a group, it is important that other group members (and possibly also other groups) are informed. It is often considered better not to inform clients who are not involved in order not to trouble them. This decision, however, is made at the expense of safety and creates a new secret, while other clients are often left with the feeling that there is something going on. It is important for them to be told what the commotion and upset are all about. If it is decided not to do so, clients will hear fragments of stories and piece them together themselves and may come up with a version of the story which is possibly more frightening than the reality.

It is not necessary to tell the other members of the group about the details of the abuse, but they should know that what has happened concerns sexual abuse or inappropriate sexual behaviour. They need to hear what is going to be done now to guarantee safety in the organisation. Will the rules be changed? And what will happen with the (suspected) perpetrator? This is important for them to know, certainly if this concerns another client or person within the organisation. It is important information because it can be (and often is) the case that the perpetrator has not only abused this one client, but has also abused other clients. It is also possible that other clients were involved in the situation or that the client who has come forward as victim also carried out sexual acts with others themselves.

If the clients experience openness about the situation, this gives them the chance to be able to tell their own story. If not personally asked, they will not often do this themselves, as they can be discouraged by the commotion which is going on around them and not want to cause additional trouble. Or they may be scared about what is going to happen if they also talk about what has taken place. Clients can suffer extremely under such secrets.

In addition, it is also possible that clients have done similar things themselves, whether or not this is only in their own eyes. In response to the events they will wonder if they will be sent away. After informing the group members, it is essential to further discuss the questions and feelings arising from the situation in individual conversations with clients.

When sexual abuse takes place in a group of people of the same age, other clients are always indirectly involved. They frequently experience the tension and the change in emotional care provided by the professional caregiver. In addition, clients can be ashamed of being part of a group in which sexual abuse has taken place and they can ask themselves how it is possible that they did not see anything. They can also feel bad because they have not been able to protect their group member. Maybe they had suspicions, but did nothing about it. Other clients often stay loyal to the person who carried out the abuse. They cannot imagine that this person could actually have done such a thing, resulting in all sorts of splitting phenomena and loyalty conflicts (see Sections 2.2.1 and 9.1.6).

Considering the prevalence figures, it is predictable that a number of the clients in the group will have a history of abuse themselves. Even if they are not involved in this particular situation, they will still be 'triggered' by the disclosure. Feelings from the past will reoccur; they re-experience the former abuse. It is possible that clients will seize this opportunity to talk about the abuse that they themselves have experienced in the past, which they have kept secret until now. It is important that clients know, hear and understand that they can talk to someone about these feelings and questions.[6]

Finally it is important to realise that the disclosure of sexual abuse can also create insecurity for clients who are sexually active themselves or who are experimenting with sexuality. It is possible that they mistakenly receive the message that all sexuality must be avoided. It is recommended to also keep an eye open for this. The topic 'healthy sexuality', which is often difficult to talk about, needs to be addressed so that clients can ask their questions on the subject.

## 5.2 The SOS programme for the client with an intellectual disability

In this section we describe the psychological first aid provided in the sessions between the professional and the victim with an intellectual disability. The first aid does not only take place in the four sessions which are described for the client. The greatest part of the recovery takes place in the other 23 hours of the day, during which the client remains in their normal surroundings. For this reason, it is important that parents, relatives and professional caregivers are well prepared for their role in this process. Preparing these people for this task takes place in the sessions that are included in this programme and begins with the support for these people themselves. When the significant people surrounding the client feel supported, experience trust and have strategies for dealing with their own reactions and those of the client, then much has already been achieved.

The first aim of the SOS programme is that people are supported in handling the initial upheaval and stress. In the last few years much research has been conducted into the way in which people's natural coping mechanisms can be optimally supported with the aim of dealing with the experience of sexual abuse in both the short and the long term.[7] One of the most important factors here is building contact and experiencing a reliable and safe relationship. Sexual abuse is a form of interpersonal violence – violence committed by one person towards another person. It is evident that this will have an effect on the way in which other relationships are experienced, not only by the victim themselves, but also in the surrounding area, by everyone who hears about it and is affected by it. This leads to distrust and fear, while at the same time, people, being social beings, always depend on one another, which creates a confusing dilemma.[8] This is of even greater influence for people with an intellectual disability, on the one hand because they are dependent on the (many) others in their relationships due to their disability, and on the other hand, certainly when they are living within a service provider, they cannot personally choose with whom they do and do not have contact. Considering this, forming a safe and healthy relationship can be a corrective experience in itself, alongside the main content of the sessions.

### 5.2.1 Attitude aspects

As previously mentioned, it is important that the professional shows a direct, sensitive and open attitude during the sessions. The professional acts as a role model for all of those involved concerning how they should respond to the situation, and at the same time, in their own behaviour, provides an example of a safe relationship. In order to do so it is important to stay calm and composed. Courage and helpfulness are essential qualities, as are visibility and approachability. It is vital that the client experiences that they are actually being seen and helped, and does not have to do everything themselves, and that other people take the initiative to do so at appropriate times and prove themselves to be trustworthy.

---

During contact, be prepared that, due to 'relational traumas', people can be defensive or otherwise behave overwhelmingly. It is important to recognise and consider both reactions as fear reactions. This can be done by creating safety, in the form of safety messages and stability in daily routines.

---

In the sessions with the client it is important that the client is stimulated to think for themselves as much as possible, to express themselves and to think of solutions. The will of victims of sexual abuse has often been broken. The victim has the tendency not to trust their own thoughts anymore, but those of the perpetrator. The perpetrator has initiated this. By focusing on thinking for themselves and showing trust in this process, the professional contributes to the client coming back into contact with their own will and their own will becoming perceptible once again.

It is the task of the professional to optimally support the client and in doing so to seek 'power moments', together with the client. These are moments in which the client has previously had to do something difficult and has been successful in doing so. This can be winning a sport competition, preparing a meal or learning to ride a bicycle. The actual activity does not matter. What is important is that, when the client thinks back, they are filled with a feeling of pride and power. This feeling can be used to give the client the courage to also bring this unpleasant, difficult time to a good end. It is important that the professional shows optimism and, as often so beautifully said, 'sows hope' of overcoming the after-effects.[9]

### 5.2.2 Preparation by the professional

Before the first session takes place, it is advisable to gather as much information as possible about the client and about what is known about the events up to now. With the help of the dossier, it is important to assess the client's developmental level regarding the different developmental areas (cognitive, social and emotional). In addition, information is needed regarding the language level and possible additional problems (psychological disorders, syndromes or other disabilities). Information about the other various developmental areas is required to determine the tempo of the sessions and to select appropriate worksheets. Information about the past history is necessary in regard to earlier traumas and possible attachment problems.

If there have been earlier experiences of sexual abuse, it is important to acquire information about the sort, prevalence and incidence of the abuse. Such information is relevant due to the fact that these events can already be, or can get, mixed up in the perception of the client. In order to recognise this, past information is necessary. Consequently, the different experiences can then be organised into 'the past' and 'the present'. Such a definition can help to make it easier to cope with the intensity of the experience.

### *Making an inventory of the symptoms*

An inventory is made of the (trauma-related) symptoms of the client. When doing so, it is important not only to consider the self-report made by the client. For people with an intellectual disability it is extremely difficult to report about themselves, apart from in the here and now. This is due to the fact that self-report requires people to see themselves from a distance, as a separate being, to make a conclusion about this, to express this in words and to report it back. This requires abstract thinking. One of the attributes of the thought processes of people with a disability is that abstract thinking is lacking or is extremely limited.

Information from the parents/relatives must be sought before the sessions, about the well-being of the client and which themes play a role. It is good to realise that people with an intellectual disability are more dependent on their surroundings than others and that people in different environments (home, living accommodation, day care centres or school) can report very different observations. It can be of value to observe which factors in the surroundings appear to increase symptoms and which support strengths.

## 5.2.3 Alignment with the internal protocols and the police

The SOS programme should be started as soon as possible after the disclosure of sexual abuse by a client. Experience and research shows that fast interventions are beneficial to the process of dealing with the abuse.[10] In organisations, a protocol is put into action after a disclosure of sexual abuse, which outlines the allocation of duties and the steps which should be made in order to make the completion of the process run as smoothly as possible. It is recommended that the SOS programme is included as part of this protocol.

In order to make an eventual (police) inquiry run as smoothly as possible, the client should be spoken with as little as possible about what has actually happened. The reason for this is to prevent the client from being influenced – consciously or unconsciously – during conversations with others and therefore eventually giving a less reliable statement. Only after giving a statement to the police (studio hearing) is it possible to openly talk to the client about the details of what has actually happened. Here lies an important point for alignment between the police and care service providers. It is clear that the principle of finding out the truth can be at odds with the principles which apply to an effective intervention after a traumatic event. This requires fast action and good co-operation (see Section 3.4.2).

It has been previously stated that the first session of the SOS programme takes place shortly after a possible minimal fact interview (see Section 1.5). At that moment, the statement for the police and the studio hearing have not yet happened and the professional, who conducts the sessions, must be aware of the importance of this. It is recommended to consult the police before the first session concerning a subsequent police report and hearing, and to inform them about the type and frequency of the interventions which the client is facing. By doing so, mutual uncertainties and misunderstanding can be eliminated and optimal agreements can be made.

In designing the sessions for the client, attention has been paid to the police establishing the truth, and questions about facts and details concerning the event(s) are explicitly not asked. For this reason, making a drawing of what has happened is sufficient to start with. Questions are not asked about the drawing, but it is used as a starting point for asking about how the client is feeling and about the side effects they are experiencing.

In later sessions, after the police process has been completed, talking about the facts and circumstances of the abuse can be functional. For example, to emphasise what the client could have done to stand their ground during the abuse situation, or how their actions have led to the abuse having now stopped.

### 5.2.4 Time and place of the sessions with the client

People with a disability strongly attach themselves to habits and do not like to break them. This is certainly the case when additional issues are present, such as autism spectrum disorders and/or complex and chronic trauma. A fixed and predictable daily routine programme contributes to a feeling of safety and helps the client to feel in control of their life. These habits form the first point of control for clients, especially after situations in which the control over their life was missing in an extreme way, such as is the case in sexual abuse. Changes in this structure bring uncertainties. Breaking a steady pattern in order to make space for the support session is a change which the client can experience as threatening. It therefore requires consideration as to how the sessions can be organised in such a way – and at a time – that creates as little disruption as possible to the anchor points which are important for the client. This is different for each client and requires knowledge about the client and alignment and consultation with the system.

It is not advised to plan sessions for children in the evening or to hold the sessions for adults later in the evening. The reason for this lies in the fact that the client needs to have time to process the information and to let it 'sink in'. It also helps if the session is not the last activity which the client does during the day and that, after the session, an activity follows in which the presence of a professional caregiver/parent/relative is normal and that daily life is continued. Experience teaches that this is difficult to provide in a group home in a (late) evening situation before the client goes to bed and is then alone.

With regard to the location, preference is given to a neutral place for people with a mild to moderate intellectual disability, where they will not be disturbed and where there are not too many stimuli. In principle, a location is chosen outside the house, because there should be more peace and privacy there, and it is also easier to realise new forms of interaction in a new situation. If the abuse took place outside the home, holding the sessions in a different location will prevent emotionally charged memories unintentionally being linked to the home situation.

Situations can also arise in which it is preferable to conduct the sessions in the home situation, for example when it is difficult for the client to make the transfer from what they have learnt in the sessions to the home situation, and when there is (too) little support to realise this in another way. Other reasons can be, for example, to be able to practise certain methods on location, such as relaxation techniques.

For people with a severe intellectual disability, the sessions should be held in the home situation in the presence of a significant other. The developmental level means that the trusted person and the trusted place form the primary starting point to benefit recovery. The emphasis of the sessions for people with a severe intellectual disability does not lie on directly working with what has happened, but on rediscovering the primary feeling of safety and contact. In this case the main aim is the experience of closeness, safety and security, and calming the dysregulation experience.

### 5.2.5 Alone or together

The question as to whether the sessions with the client should take place with the client alone, or together with a trusted other, is assessed per client. For some clients, an individual conversation with a professional can be advantageous, as this recognises their autonomy and appeals more strongly to their personal thought process. For others, the presence of a trusted other is essential. It is up to the practitioner, together with the parents/relatives and professional caregivers, to assess which is best and/or to inform the client about the decision. As a rule, when the developmental level of the client is lessening, the choice is increasingly made for the presence of the significant other. It is also important to consider to what extent the professional fulfils the role of trusted person.

#### *Trusted person*

If the choice is made for the presence of the trusted person, it is important that, when choosing who this person will be, the resilience of the person themselves is taken into consideration and whether or not they will be able to actually be there for the client. This requires the person to be further along in the process of dealing with the abuse themselves and to be able to stay in control at the moments at which memories are triggered during the session. In addition, it is very disturbing to witness the full upheaval and fear of someone with whom you have a strong connection, as can happen during the sessions. It is necessary to pay attention to these issues, both before and after the sessions.

Furthermore, when choosing a trusted person, it is important that someone is found who can provide space for the personal thoughts and will-process described above which must be set in motion again; the trusted person must be able to position themselves in the background. This seems obvious, but experience teaches that in the daily support of people with a disability, as a result of organisational and institutionalised patterns, there is actually little space for this attitude. It can be difficult for both parties to suddenly change a pattern of interaction which has sometimes been built up and relied on over many years.

Finally, when considering who will be present at the session, it is important to pay attention to the situation in which the abuse took place. It can occur that a one-to-one situation in a room can act as a trigger and can therefore be experienced as threatening, in such a way that the abuse is somehow re-experienced. In such a situation it is obviously important to make sure that a trusted third person is present.

### 5.2.6 Preparing the client

Not only must the professional be prepared, but attention must also be paid to preparation for the client. The client (of a moderate or mild intellectual level of disability) is invited to come and talk about how they are feeling and to learn about how they can start to feel better. The client can be told that they will be able to express all of their questions and concerns during the sessions and that the aim is to help them as much as possible.

It is important that the person who prepares the client can answer questions about the practical aspects concerning the help sessions, for example when the sessions will take place, where they will be, how long they will last, who will be going with them and how missing the regular activities will be organised. If the client has not yet met the professional, then it is important that the person who helps prepare the client for the session expresses the fact that the professional is a pleasant person. A photo of the professional can possibly help in the preparation. A short 'meet and greet' can be arranged beforehand, in which the professional visits and introduces themselves.

### 5.2.7 Resistance from the client

Some clients show resistance to the help offered. This often derives from fear, uncertainty and mistrust resulting from their history and/or what they have recently experienced. In this case, good explanation and reassurance will help.

It is also possible that the client, due to their concrete level of perception, cannot imagine the fact that the present symptoms can be related to and are all about what they have experienced. For these clients, simple psychoeducation in relation to this subject is appropriate. It can also help to encourage the client to express all of their doubts to the professional, and the presence of a known support person is then recommended at the first session.

When visiting the professional appears to be a step too far, the professional can choose to visit the client at home for the first session. The first session should focus on building a relationship and relieving symptoms which are sometimes very concrete and practical. If this step also prompts too much resistance, a model can be chosen in which the personal caregiver or another trusted figure, who has been instructed in a 'train the trainer' model, help the client as much as possible. In such a situation it is probable that further psychological evaluation and treatment will be urgently required.

### 5.2.8 Structure of the session

In the implementation of the SOS programme, the professional must realise that there is not a readymade content for the conversations which can be followed as a standard procedure. In order to increase the feeling of safety and for the client to be able to deal with what has happened, a fixed sequence is advised during the sessions.

Start the first session by determining the 'rules' and what is going to be done in the sessions, and continue to follow the same order. The course of the session can also be determined and visualised by using a comic strip story or pictograms, depending on which form suits the client best.

Which subject is addressed at which moment depends on the individual situation. Subjects can be clustered into three main themes which are part of every session:

- talking about sexual abuse
- emotional support for the parents
- providing psychoeducation.

When talking about the sexual abuse, the professional gives the client the opportunity to reconstruct and to order their experiences. Emotional support is given by providing a listening ear and by being there in a time of upheaval. Naming, discussing and giving meaning to thoughts and feelings which the client is experiencing regarding the abuse is essential. Providing psychoeducation is a central part of the SOS programme. By providing information (adapted to their level) about trauma and dealing with trauma and about stress reactions and how to deal with them, clients will gain understanding, control and a feeling of certainty of being able to deal with the situation.

During the structure of the sessions, attention should be paid to the principle of the 'cognitive affective cognitive sandwich' (see Box 5.1). This describes the importance of surrounding emotionally charged issues with more structured and thought-directed issues and aims, so that the emotion remains manageable for the client. Always finish with less emotive issues, so that the client leaves in a lessened emotional state.

### Box 5.1 Framework: sandwich technique

An example of the sandwich technique can be seen in the structure of session 1 for people with a moderate intellectual disability (see Section 5.3.1). After the introduction, a more cognitive part is started in the form of psychoeducation, about how symptoms can arise after abuse and how important it is to talk about these. Subsequently the more emotional part starts, in which the personal after-effects are explored. Then something calming follows: considering what is appropriate to say to people about the abuse in a cognitive way. The session is rounded off with a relaxation technique, after which the caregiver is present and a cognitive summary is made of how to continue the process and what has been done so far.

## 5.2.9 Using the help book

When starting the SOS programme, a help book is made for and with the client. This consists of a folder with a loose-leaf system.

This folder can be adapted to the functional level, problem areas and themes which apply to the specific client. Depending on these points, the professional selects work forms which suit the client, along the way and per session, and these act as a foundation from which to 'discuss' the sexual abuse and the effects of it.

The work forms are divided into trauma-related themes: safety, worries, pain, fear, anger, relaxation and perspective.[11] For each theme, work forms are provided for various levels of cognitive functioning: mild, moderate and severe intellectual disability.

Alongside the work forms, information sheets are given which can be used in the psychoeducation around sexual abuse and dealing with trauma, but also (if applicable) for providing information about giving a police statement. The drawings which the client makes during the sessions are also included in the help book.

Additionally, the help book can be used as a sort of diary in which the client and the professional caregivers and parents/relatives make notes about what the positive and less positive things are which are being experienced. Furthermore, the help book is used as a form of communication between the client, the practitioner, the professional caregivers and parents/relatives regarding the progress of the sessions and the transfer of what they have learnt to daily life.

For people with a more severe intellectual disability, the help book will be of less use for the client themselves and will fulfil a function as a form of communication between significant people in the surrounding system and as an observation and registration method about the well-being of the client (see Chapter 7).

## 5.3 Client sessions

The professional organises four sessions for the client. The first contact moment is as soon as possible, preferably within a week after the disclosure/discovery takes place (and after the minimal fact interview). The second session takes place approximately a week later. The third session is a combined session, in which the client, their family system and the healthcare professionals involved share their experiences, and (learn to) communicate with each other about what has happened. This combined session is planned approximately one month after the start of the programme.

A follow-up session is held for the various healthcare professionals after eight weeks.

In the following paragraphs, the four support sessions for the client are described as they can generally be held. The sessions are not meant as a fixed method, but aim to serve as an example and as inspiration. It is important that the professional adapts the session for the client in advance by adding theme and subjects from the client's immediate environment. Work forms must be chosen which suit the functional level and interests of the client. This can mean that drawing paper is not used, but that instead the computer is used for an important part of the session or that music is added to the session.

For people with a severe intellectual disability, depending on the additional disabilities, greater adaptations will often be necessary. For ideas on this subject see Chapter 7. Here, work forms for clients with a severe intellectual disability are described. In Chapter 6, work forms are described for people with a mild and moderate intellectual disability.

### 5.3.1 Client session 1: as soon as possible

What is needed?

- SOS handbook
- Help book for client
- Drawing equipment
- Appropriate worksheets, for example:
    - 'What has happened?' (Section 6.3)
    - 'How am I doing?' (Section 6.3)
    - 'Where does that strange feeling come from?' (Section 6.3)
    - 'What is bothering you?' (Section 6.3)
    - 'Relaxation exercises' (Section 6.3)
    - 'How do I tell others about it?' (Section 6.3).

Duration of the session: 45 minutes.

### *Introduction*

Get to know the client briefly and explain what is going to happen: how often, where and when we will meet and how are we going to meet? The help book is given to the client, explaining that you will write and draw in the book about what you talk about together, so that the client can look back at everything at home if they need to.

### *Talking about the sexual abuse*

*'We are here together because you have experienced some very unpleasant things. Everyone reacts differently to things that have happened to them. Some people get scared, others get angry or have to cry a lot. How do you feel? Let's make a drawing of what has happened.'*

### *Psychoeducation on stress reactions and dealing with trauma*

*'If you have experienced unpleasant things, you will often feel bad. Sometimes you will be sad, angry, scared, guilty, ashamed or you can have other feelings. Sometimes there are so many feelings that you don't know what you feel anymore.*

*'How do you feel? Draw what you look like with all the different feelings. What do you think about when you feel like that?*

*'If you have experienced unpleasant things, you have to think about them a lot. This often happens when it's quiet and you haven't got anything to do; for example, at school or at your workplace when it's quiet, when you watch TV or when you go to sleep. Sometimes you see what has happened like a film in your head. Sometimes you have frightening dreams or nightmares.*

*'Sometimes you see, hear or feel something that seems like what you have experienced. This shocks you a lot. It seems as if it can happen again. Sometimes, you don't know the difference between what is real and what seems to be real. That makes you scared! Then it helps to ask the caregivers or your parents whether or not what you are feeling is real or whether it just seems like what you have experienced.*

*'Some people don't want to talk about it or think about it. They don't want to have anything to do with it. That's almost impossible, because you automatically keep thinking about it. A lot of people are startled quicker or get angry easily. Sleeping can also be difficult. You can get a stomach ache or headache or get really busy or lazy*

*and tired. Some people think that they have become strange and are scared that they are going mad. But that is not true. It is normal and common that you feel like this. It is because of what you have experienced. And you will find that it ends after a while. Then you'll feel normal again.'*

## *Support and making an inventory of symptoms*

*'Maybe you are also very scared, or you are startled quickly or you see images of what has happened, or you have bad dreams. It is different for everyone. Shall we see what is bothering you and what is not bothering you?'*

Fill in the worksheet 'What is bothering you?' together (or make a drawing) and if necessary help the client by including information that you have received from the parents and professional caregivers.

With the worksheet as starting point, you and the client can look at what could help them with their specific after-effects. One idea is to take a piece of paper per symptom and write the symptom on it. Another idea is to make a drawing (not too big) of the symptom and to write underneath it what helps. This can also be done in the form of pictograms/pictures.

If there are a large number of symptoms, it is sometimes possible to combine several of the symptoms, or to ask the client what the most important/worse things are and where you should begin.

*'Things that can help are, for example, talking about it with one of the professional caregivers, looking for something to take your mind off it (playing a computer game, listening to music, watching television, not sitting on your own in your room but going to the living room, doing something with somebody else, doing sports, dancing and jumping up and down). And, of course, looking after yourself; spoiling yourself a bit is also fine.*

*'What doesn't help is doing things such as not going to your work or not doing fun activities because you feel bad and tired. It is actually important to do these things. Drinking lots of beer or breezers or taking drugs is not a good idea. That might seem to help for a while, but later you'll feel even worse.'*

### *Relaxation techniques*

*'A relaxation technique can help when you feel bad. Shall we try this?'* (See Section 6.3, Relaxation exercises.)

Do the relaxation technique together and explain that the more often you do this, the better it will go. Agree with the professional caregivers that they support the client in their daily practice.

If necessary, prepare the police interview (after consultation with the police). Prepare the client for the police interview, if that is yet to take place, and if the date falls between the first and second session.

### *The end of the session – who do you want to talk to and what can you say?*

*'Sometimes it's difficult to think of what you should say to somebody about what has happened. But it is still good to talk about it. You haven't done anything wrong and if you don't feel well it is important that people know why you're feeling that way. Then they can understand and help you better. What could you say to them?'*

Help the client to think of a suitable text for various people. At work, at school and with possible group members, the client could say that they have experienced something awful (in the area of sexuality) and that's why they don't feel well. For good friends, a slightly more extensive text may be appropriate. For this purpose you can use the worksheet: 'How do I tell others about it?' (see Section 6.3).

Ask the client if they would prefer to tell other people about it themselves, or if they would rather do this together with somebody else. It is also possible that a client would prefer someone else to talk about it. In that case, attention should be paid to the moment when the client next sees that person. If the client chooses one of the last two options, arrange this with the person who comes to collect the client.

Rounding off the session is clearly described. Let the client describe what has been done and what they found the most fun and the least fun today, and what they thought was the best thing. This allows you to find out what someone has remembered and how it has come across to the client. Write in the notebook (or let the client write) what has been discussed.

Make sure that the relaxation technique, the list of symptoms and what helps are included in the help book and give this book to the client. Add blank pages on which the client and/or significant others can write or draw their actions, feelings and questions. Agree on the best place for the client to keep the book, so that they can find it quickly if they need to. Agree that the client brings the book with them next time.

Discuss with the client what is going to be told to the professional caregiver/parent who is coming to collect the client. Include the professional caregiver/parent in the last five minutes of the session and discuss in short what has happened during the session. Ask this person to help the client in using the help book and possibly also do the relaxation techniques together. If the client wishes, agree on who (separately or together with the client) will be told about what has happened.

Give the client a big compliment. Tell the client again when the next session will take place.

If the client's pace is very slow, the relaxation technique part can be left out and you can choose to make a help plan for fewer after-effects (or for just one: feeling bad).

### 5.3.2 Client session 2: after one week

What is needed?

- SOS handbook
- Help book for client
- Drawing equipment
- Appropriate worksheets, for example:
    - 'What has happened?' (Section 6.3)
    - 'How am I doing?' (Section 6.3)
    - 'What is bothering you?' (Section 6.3)
    - 'Relaxation exercises' (Section 6.3)
    - Preparation from joint session.

Duration of the session: 45 minutes.

### *Talking about the sexual abuse*

Start by asking how the week went. What has the client experienced during the week? Talk about the negative aspects and also ask about pleasant, enjoyable experiences. Has anything else happened which has got something to do with the abuse? How have others reacted to hearing about the abuse? What have other clients, parents, family and professional caregivers said? What went well and what was less enjoyable? Possibly fill in the worksheet 'What has happened?' (see Section 6.3).

### *Psychoeducation on stress reactions and support needs*

Use the help book and discuss the after-effects of the abuse, for example using the worksheet 'How am I doing?' (see Section 6.3). Which symptoms are the client experiencing now? Is the client visualising images of the abuse? Are there things that remind him/her about it? Ask about the symptoms, one at a time. Discuss with the client whether or not they have done the things discussed and written down under the heading 'What helps?' in the first session.

Ask which activities the client has tried to do and which did and didn't help. If something didn't help, ask how the activity was done. Consider whether the instructions need to be explained again. When instructions are not followed properly, this is often due to the fact that the client and the professional caregivers have not understood them clearly enough. Has the client already experienced small positive changes? What is going better now compared to last week?

Emphasise activities which have helped, if this is a safe and good way to deal with the after-effects (adequate coping). Encourage the client to do these activities more often. When coping strategies are less effective (for example, if someone stays awake all night playing computer games to prevent themselves from having nightmares), then look for other ways to deal with negative feelings and stress, for example relaxation techniques.

### *Relaxation techniques*

*'A relaxation technique can help when you feel bad. Shall we try this?'* (See Section 6.3, Relaxation exercises.)

Do the relaxation technique together and explain that the more often you do this, the better it will go. Agree with the professional caregivers that they support the client in their daily practice.

If necessary, prepare the police interview (after consultation with the police). Prepare the client for the police interview, if that is yet to take place, and if the date falls between the second and fourth session.

### *Preparing the joint session*

In the second session the client will be prepared for the joint session. Tell the client that the next session will be held together with the parents/family:

*'Next time we will all talk with each other about what has happened. This is important because everyone has been shocked by what has happened. By talking about it together, we can help each other. We can also tell your parents and family how they can help you in the best way.'*

Explain the structure of the next session in concrete terms:

*'We will meet on...at...together in room... We will have a cup of coffee or tea and a biscuit. I (or the name of someone else) will lead the conversation and make sure that it will be a good conversation.'*

Prepare the third session by using the following questions:

*'Which of the professional caregivers would you like to be present at the session? And which parent/family members? Who is good at helping you? And why? What could you say about what has happened? What is important for you? What would you like to ask or hear from the caregivers and your family?'*

And:

*'Are there other things which you find important to talk about during the conversation?'*

It is important to actively think about things together with the client and to suggest things. It is possible that the client will want to hear from the parents and caregivers that they are also greatly shocked and that they do not think that it is the client's fault. It is also possible that the caregivers feel bad and think that they should have paid more attention. Maybe the client had tried to warn them by giving signals, or in their own eyes had tried to tell others about it but the message didn't come across clearly. The client can tell others this and parents and professional caregivers can tell the client that they take this very seriously and that they will behave differently in the future.

Maybe there are practical things which the client would like to have, such as a different room, or rearranging the room in such a way that the client is not constantly reminded of what has happened. Doing extra activities can help as a distraction, or maybe the client would like someone to accompany them during activities which the client would prefer not to do alone at the moment. The client might like to talk about other things which will help to them to feel safer.

Also discuss the after-effects of the abuse and how the parents or professionals can help them deal with these.

*'When we have finished talking, we will do the "We stand strong together" activity. At the end of the session this will be yours and you can keep it in a place which you think is suitable.*

*'At the end of the conversation we will tell each other what we thought of the session and if we need to talk to each other separately. Then we will eat and/or drink something together and afterwards carry on with the normal activities for that day.'*

### *The end of the session*

State clearly that the session has ended and ask how the client experienced it. Let the client describe what has been done and what they found the most fun and the least fun today, and what they thought was the best thing. This allows you to find out what they have remembered and how it has come across to the client. Write in the notebook (or let the client write) what has been discussed. Also write down the preparation for the combined session in the book.

The help book is given to the client to take home with them. Agree that the client will bring the book with them to the session next week and that they can use it during the joint conversation.

Discuss with the client what is going to be told to the caregiver/parent, who is coming to collect the client. Include the caregiver/parent in the last five minutes of the session and discuss in short what has happened during the session. Give the client a big compliment and ask the caregiver to help the client in using the help book and possibly also do the relaxation techniques together. Tell the client again when the next session will take place.

### 5.3.3 Client session 3: the joint session – after three weeks

What is needed?

- SOS handbook
- Help book for client
- The presence of the manager/team leader as co-support during the conversation
- Coffee/tea and a biscuit
- Flip-chart, whiteboard or something similar
- Worksheets 'Together we are strong', for example:
    - 'Together we are strong – the plaster' (Section 6.3)
    - 'Together we are strong – the message' (Section 6.3)
    - 'Together we are strong – the song' (Section 6.3).
- Materials with which to make the chosen 'Together we are strong' activity, such as drawing and craft equipment. Depending on the client's personal taste you can also use glitter, stars, photos, a computer and so on.

Duration of the session: approximately two hours in total.

---

Joint discussion: one hour. Afterwards an informal session is held with everyone present, which aims to create a feeling of togetherness, clear communication and getting back to normal life again.

---

#### *Talking about the sexual abuse*

Tell those involved about the session.

*'Today we're going to talk about what has happened. That is important because everyone is shocked by what has happened. By talking about it together we can help each other.'*

Describe the structure of the session clearly:

*'We are here together in…'s room. We will begin by drinking a cup of tea or coffee with a biscuit. I (or the name of someone else) will lead the discussion and make sure that it goes well. When we have finished talking, we will make something together. After that we will talk some more, then we will proceed with ending the session together.'*

Give a short description of what has happened. If the police interview has already been held, then it will be possible to say more than when it has yet to take place. It is possible to use a timeline and/or sociogram to tell the story.

### *Psychoeducation on stress reactions and support needs*

Subsequently the psychoeducation part of the session takes place:

*'Everyone is very shocked by what has happened and each person reacts in their own way. You may be angry, scared or sad. Let's hear how everyone has reacted.'*

The person who leads the conversation then gives those present, one at a time, the chance to tell how they have reacted and this is written on the flip-chart. For clients who cannot read or write you can work with smileys to communicate the reactions of those involved.

It is important that the reactions of parents and professional caregivers are prepared during previous meetings. The joint session is intended as a support session for the client. Positive actions and characteristics of the client should be mentioned, such as how well the client is coping even though something awful has happened. This can be done, for example, by saying: *'I reacted in an angry/scared way'* and then telling the client:

*'You did well to tell others about it (if this is how it has been discovered) and how you are dealing with it now. It is not your fault that I'm feeling like this. It is the perpetrator's fault, they were at fault. Not you.'*

It is important to steer the content of the discussion in this direction and, if necessary, to add this information yourself. Clients must be relieved of guilt and must be empowered! If other participants in the discussion require extra support, this should take place at a different moment.

### *Together we are strong!*

The client is asked how they are feeling now and if there is anything else they would like to say. The person who led the discussion with the client in session 2 helps the client (if necessary using the help book) to express what is on their mind. Attention is paid to practical issues, safety and reactions to what parents and professionals have said. In addition, attention is paid to the wishes of the client regarding the type of support during the next few weeks. What is the best way to help the client and with which activities? What does the client like doing and what helps best?

The 'Together we are strong' activity is meant to break through the isolation which people can feel after experiencing something traumatic. Above all, it is meant to let clients experience that everyone is working together and help to make dealing with the abuse bearable. The most appropriate 'Together we are strong' activity is chosen beforehand:

- 'Together we are strong – the plaster' (Box 5.2 and Section 6.3)
- 'Together we are strong – the message' (Section 6.3)
- 'Together we are strong – the song' (Section 6.3)
- 'Together we are strong – music' (Section 7.4).

---

## Box 5.2 Framework – the plaster

For this 'Together we are strong' activity, a thick piece of paper or thin cardboard is needed, on which the professional has drawn a big plaster (see Section 6.3). The professional introduces the method and explains in a way which is suited to the level of the client that abuse hurts:

*'It is not exactly the same as having a wound on your body, but it is the same sort of thing. When you have a wound on your body, you stick a plaster on it. That helps to let it heal more quickly. The plaster keeps the dirt out and protects the wound, also if you bump into something. If your feelings have been wounded (or your heart or your spirit or whatever you would like to call it) then you can't stick a real plaster on it. But what we can do is make a beautiful plaster for the wound together. You can hang this plaster up in your (bed) room. You can look at it whenever you feel bad. Then you'll remember that we are all supporting and helping you and that we want to give you the plaster so*

*that you'll feel less pain. We're going to make the plaster as beautiful as possible together and decorate it so that it will really suit you!'*

Then everyone joins in decorating the plaster. The plaster should be drawn large enough for everyone to be able to work on it at the same time. During the process, the client is asked what they think of it: if they like the colours, the pictures and so on. While working, those present make positive statements about the characteristics of the client. The plaster is finished when it has been coloured in completely and the client is happy with it. When it is finished, tell the client again why the plaster has been made. It is also possible to hang the plaster up together in the room afterwards.

### *The end of the session – talking about what we thought of the discussion*

Here you can choose to do this with everyone involved or only with the client. The choice depends on how the discussion goes, the characteristics of the client and of the parents (are there problems relating to the parents, are there intense emotions and so on?). Can the client talk about this with the other people present or will the client benefit more from talking about it individually with you? Write in the client's help book (or let the client write) about the conversation and what they thought of it. Put the joint activity, or a photo of it, in the client's help book and let them take it home with them.

### *What next?*

Agree and write down who will support the client in the following weeks and at which times. Tell the client that these people are going to support them and that the client doesn't have to visit the professional during the next few weeks. Say that an appointment will be made after a while to see how the client is feeling and how they are being supported. Make an actual appointment and write this down in the help book.

## 5.3.4 Client session 4: follow-up – after two months

After two months, the client will visit the behavior specialist for the last time in the psychological first aid sessions. The client brings the help book with them, in which they, the parents and the professional caregivers, have made a record of how the client has been since the joint session and the 'Together we are strong' session.

What is needed?

- SOS handbook
- Help book for client
- Drawing equipment
- Appropriate worksheets, for example:
  - 'What has happened?' (Section 6.3)
  - 'How am I doing?' (Section 6.3).

Duration of the session: 45 minutes.

### *Talking about the sexual abuse*

Talk to the client about what has happened since the joint session. If a statement has been made, it is possible that the hearing (and other research) has been carried out by the police. Pay attention to this experience and, if necessary, use the worksheet 'What has happened?' (see Section 6.3).

### *Psychoeducation on stress reactions and support needs*

*'Shall we talk about how you have been feeling?'*

Fill in the worksheet 'How am I doing?'(Section 6.3) together and, if necessary, help the client by providing information, which you have received beforehand from the parents and professional caregivers.

Using the help book, look back to how the client was feeling during the first session. Compare the feelings experienced then and now and emphasise the improvement, if things are actually going better now. Say that this is good news and that, as time goes by, it will continue to improve. Say that the client has worked hard to achieve this, that they deserve respect and can be proud of themselves. Emphasise the client's strength in dealing with the situation.

If there seems to be no difference in how the client is feeling between the first session and the present, then it is important to talk to the client about why this is. Describe how dealing with such experiences goes in ups and downs, and that the client will continue to receive support in dealing with the situation. Compare it, for example, to learning to ride a bicycle: *'Do you remember learning to ride a bicycle? How did that go the first time?'* The client will probably say that it didn't go very well and that they had to be held, or they fell over, or something similar. Ask how cycling goes now. The client will probably say that they don't need help anymore. Subsequently you can say that dealing with sexual abuse works in kind of the same way. It has to be practised and it takes some time, but then it is possible to learn to deal with it.

### *Is further help necessary?*

Whether or not further help is needed is discussed. This depends on what the client says and what the parents/relatives and professional caregivers report back. Further help can be necessary if the symptoms do not lessen (enough) and the client continues to experience suffering. In the case of extremely frightened clients who demonstrate primary attachment behaviour, professional help regarding attachment and trust is indicated. Experience teaches that, in a successful therapeutic process, such behaviour will gradually lessen and be replaced by behaviour which is more appropriate to the (developmental) age.

Furthermore, it is important to offer therapeutic support to clients who – with an aim towards fulfilling their basic needs – indiscriminately orientate themselves towards others, making them extremely vulnerable to new abuse situations in the future.

If further help is needed in future, it is important for the professional to be able to tell the client how this will take place and what the client can expect.

### *The end of the session and evaluation*

Finally, using the help book, the client and professional look back together at the sessions and talk about what did and didn't go well and what did and didn't work. Clients are often able to express in their own way what was beneficial and what didn't help. It is important to write down the things that the client described as being helpful in the help book. The client can also make a drawing of these. These notes and drawings are intended for the client themselves, so that they can later look back at them in the help book – this is definitely a good thing to do at moments in which the client isn't feeling well. Professional caregivers and parents can also look back through the book if they need to.

The session ends by talking, together with the professional caregiver, about the things that have helped the client and expressing the feeling that you think that they are able to deal with the situation themselves. Thank the client for their trust and wish them all the best in the future. Tell them that you will come and visit them in the group after a while to see how things are going (and do actually do this!).

## SUMMARY

Sexual abuse has consequences for the client themselves and for people in their immediate surroundings. In this chapter, the psychological first aid for the client has been described as an essential part of the SOS programme. Various core aspects have been covered. Concentrating on safety is the first aim.

People with an intellectual disability react to sexual abuse in very different ways, depending on their history. It is important that professional caregivers are aware of what the diverse reactions can imply in light of the abuse and that they remain calm in the case of challenging behaviour. The importance of informing other clients is also mentioned.

Furthermore, general aspects are described, which can be of importance for the professional during the sessions with the client. Four sessions are described, detailing the three important themes: talking about sexual abuse, providing emotional support and psychoeducation. These sessions are intended for people with a moderate to mild intellectual disability. Psychological first aid support for people with a severe intellectual disability is further described in Chapter 7.

Chapter 6

# HELP BOOK FOR PEOPLE WITH A MILD OR MODERATE INTELLECTUAL DISABILITY

## Introduction

People with a mild to moderate intellectual disability react in different ways after suffering sexual abuse. The differences in behaviour can be explained by the developmental stage at which the person functions, combined with their previous experiences. When the perpetrator is a person who is important in the life of the client and whom the client depends on, the client's basic trust is damaged. They realise that the person on whom they rely is also the person who can hurt them. This causes confusion, distrust, helplessness, and a series of after-effects, which are also seen in people without an intellectual disability.

Psychological support after sexual abuse for this group of people focuses on the following areas: providing information and psychoeducation; relieving and making an inventory of concerns; creating safety; helping the client to order their experiences and feelings; dealing with overwhelming emotions; relaxation techniques and creating tools for survival. Exercises are provided for these topics. The exercises can be adapted or added to, depending on the client and their situation. After the session, the worksheets are added to the help book and given to the client to take home with them.

## 6.1 Core aspects for the psychological support of people with a mild intellectual disability

### 6.1.1 People with a mild intellectual disability

A mild intellectual disability indicates an IQ of between 50 and 85. In the Netherlands, an official distinction is made within this group between:

- the group with an IQ indication between 50 and 70
- the group with an IQ indication between 70 and 85.

In this book we have chosen to refer to these two groups as one group, and to refer to them as people with a mild intellectual disability. The reason for doing so is that, in practice, both groups use – and benefit from – the same method of treatment. People from these two subgroups are often comparable, due to additional issues in personal development.

People in the target group 'mild intellectual disability' are very diverse, just as is the case with those with a moderate or severe intellectual disability. People are diagnosed with a mild intellectual disability when their developmental level is between approximately 7 and 12 years. When you consider the enormous differences in development between people in this period of their lives, it becomes clear that it is impossible to generalise. For example, a conscientious school child is usually eager to conform, while a young teenager will often rebel against any form of authority.

When working with people with a mild intellectual disability within the SOS programme, it is also important to consider the substantial differences that can exist between cognitive and emotional functioning. After-effects and experiences that are seen in people with a lower level of cognitive functioning are also apparent in these people. In this case it is recommended that the interventions are adapted to the level of emotional functioning, while the design of the sessions remains in accordance with the calendar age and level of cognitive functioning.

In general, people consider those with a mild intellectual disability to display the same psychological disorders and symptoms as people without an intellectual disability.[1] After sexual abuse the same consequences are also generally seen.[2] Critics of this opinion point to the way in which differences in after-effects developing must be considered in the symptoms for people with a mild intellectual disability. The reasons for these differences are diverse, and span biological, psychological and environmental factors. Biological differences are, for example, genetic impediments. An example of psychological differences is feeling less competent. Typical environmental factors are deprivation and isolation. Emotional development and personality development generally stagnate at the level of a school child. This means that these people continue to feel dependent on significant others and do not become fully autonomous.[3]

In the psychosocial development of people with a mild intellectual disability, a distinction can be made between the cognitive, social and emotional aspect. The various aspects influence each other greatly.

### *The cognitive aspect*

The thought processes of a person with a mild intellectual disability can create both possibilities and limitations. Language is used, and it is therefore easier to communicate with them than with someone with a moderate intellectual disability. In general, school skills such as reading and writing are present, up to a maximum level of year 5 of primary school. They can talk about concrete situations. People with a mild intellectual disability learn from concrete experiences and from example. These people have problems with abstract thought and understanding complex messages and situations.

### *The social aspect*

With regard to the social aspect, it is generally the case that many of these people mainly feel connected to significant others and are loyal towards them. There is a great need for rules – and conforming to rules – concerning the immediate environment, although they tend to disobey them. The feeling of social responsibility is generally weak.

### *The emotional aspect*

In emotional perspective, people with a mild intellectual disability generally wish to be accepted and feel competent. A sense of belonging is very important. There is little perception of the future; the past determines the emotional life in the here and now.

With regard to the development of personality, the ego is still greatly dependant on the judgement of others and people are strongly attached to rules. The development of conscience is closely related to cognitive and emotional development. People can display feelings of omnipotence, or have a great need to manage skills and life.

People with a mild intellectual disability generally have restricted control over their impulses and are less able to display empathy and guilt, because they are, in cognitive terms, not (yet) able to empathise with others. Emotions such as anger, fear and happiness have usually been developed. Fury and aggression, directed at significant people, can be displayed.

### 6.1.2 Sexual abuse and people with a mild intellectual disability

When sexual abuse occurs concerning these clients, the experience will be connected to issues with authority, crossing the given boundary and the rules. Sexual abuse will be experienced as breaking the fragile autonomy of the client.

Sexual abuse means that the client's boundary has not been respected. The client will feel powerless. Fear regarding those who are stronger and older often develops, as well as sensitivity towards authority. This is connected with a basic uncertainty about personal power and capacity for protection.

The aggression which is repressed in regard to the stronger party will grow within the client and can become a source of aggression and conflict in the future. For others, the abuse will be experienced as a serious breach of privacy and the client can react with prudishness and fear of sexuality.

Feelings of guilt can be intense, because sexual abuse can also be felt as an indication for the desire to be attractive which, partly due to the disability, is an uncertain factor. This creates confusion: the sexual abuse is experienced as being negative and positive at the same time. In addition, the emotional phase of development results in an increased wish to feel competent, which relates adversely to being a victim.

Sexual abuse is mainly perpetrated by men. The consequences are diverse and depend on the sex of the client. Due to identifying with the aggressor, boys will run the risk of becoming perpetrators themselves. Girls, by identifying with the aggressor, will run the risk of developing an ambivalent attitude towards men. This can influence their choice of partner and the amount and way in which they are able to share intimacy with this partner. Due to the fact that sexual abuse is mainly caused by men, and because physical strength plays a deciding role, sexual abuse can also result in fear for their own limited personal strength.

## 6.2 Core aspects in the psychological support of people with a moderate intellectual disability

### 6.2.1 People with a moderate intellectual disability

People with a moderate intellectual disability are indicated by an IQ of between 35 and 50. This target group is very diverse. People with a moderate intellectual disability have a developmental level of between approximately four and seven years. When considering the enormous differences in development of people of this period of their lives, it becomes clear that it is impossible to generalise. For example, a headstrong and enterprising toddler differs greatly from a conscientious school child who is eager to conform.

When working with people with a moderate intellectual disability within the SOS programme, it is also important to consider possible additional issues concerning the damage of the central nervous system. In comparison with people with a mild intellectual disability, functional disorders occur relatively often, such as epilepsy, speech impairments and problems with regulating affect and aggression, as well as genetic impediments and associated behaviour phenotypes. Consideration is required of the influence of these problems in dealing with sexual abuse.

In the psychosocial development of people with a moderate intellectual disability a distinction can be made between the cognitive, social and emotional aspects. The various aspects influence each other greatly.

### *The cognitive aspect*

The thought processes of a person with a moderate intellectual disability can create possibilities and limitations. Language is used and it is therefore easier to communicate with them than with someone with a severe intellectual disability. Language is used to communicate concrete messages, and thought has a concrete character. Thought is connected to concrete situations and experiences. Thinking ahead, thinking of solutions in one's head and 'trying things out', separately from the tangible reality, is virtually impossible.

People with a moderate intellectual disability learn by experience and by example. It is difficult for them to empathise with others as their thought processes are strongly egocentric.

### *The social aspect*

With regard to the social aspect, it can be said that these people focus primarily on their immediate surroundings. The family of origin is of great influence and meaning. People with moderate intellectual disabilities have few permanent friendships, but like to socialise with people of the same age and participate in activities together. People generally feel a connection with the significant other and identify with them.

### *The emotional aspect*

From an emotional perspective, there can be feelings of omnipotence and an increased need to manage skills and life. People with a moderate intellectual disability generally have restricted control over their impulses and are less able to display empathy and guilt, because they are, in cognitive terms, not (yet) able to empathise with others. Emotions such as anger, fear, happiness and sadness have usually been developed. Anger and aggression, directed at significant people, can be displayed.

When considering the development of personality in these people, the ego is usually fragile and dependant. There is a beginning development of conscience, which initially causes confusion, in combination with the limited ability to think about cause and effect. This can be seen at moments in which the client feels guilty or over-responsible for situations which do not concern them, or underestimates their own role in a situation and shows no responsibility, when in the eyes of others this would have been considered appropriate.

### 6.2.2 Sexual abuse and people with a moderate intellectual disability

When sexual abuse takes place with these clients and the perpetrator is a significant other on whom the client is dependant, there is a large chance that the client will be damaged in their basic ability to experience trust. The need for protection, which the client displays in both a physical and an emotional way, becomes problematic. The client will experience a feeling of uncertainty about the type of emotional protection which can be expected. The client will have the tendency to avoid emotional contact instead of initiating or answering it. Due to this closed and defensive behaviour, the client will stand the chance of becoming isolated.

After sexual abuse, the client will also become confused about taking initiatives of a physical nature. They will display the tendency to give these initiatives a sexual tint and will stand the risk of being labelled as sexually challenging or solicitous.[4]

It is also possible that the client will display the opposite reaction, and become seriously inhibited and defensive. Feelings of guilt can easily develop as a consequence of the fact that the client sees themselves as being an initiator of the sexual abuse, whether or not this feeling has been fuelled by the perpetrator. Additionally, the client cannot yet master cause-and-effect relations adequately in cognitive terms.

Clients with a moderate intellectual disability, when made a victim of sexual abuse, often have a very negative judgement about what 'they have done'. Seen from the stage of emotional development in which one often feels more in control of the situation than they actually are, there is a tendency to take responsibility for what has happened (see Chapter 4).

## 6.3 The help book for people with a mild and moderate intellectual disability

The sessions described in the SOS programme for people with a mild to moderate intellectual disability are aimed at ordering the experiences and dealing with the feelings, questions and symptoms which the client experiences. Due to the fact that the differences between people with a mild intellectual disability and the differences between developmental areas can be so great, the help book should be adapted according to the needs of each individual person.

The exercises are divided into themes (safety, worries, hurt, fear, anger, relaxation and survival) and can be chosen according to what is happening in the life of the client and what is considered to be appropriate for them. The compilation of the help book and the choice of exercises therefore depend on the client's individual circumstances. There is no fixed content in the help book; this would not do justice to the many different situations which one encounters in real life.

The professional can use a folder with various tab pages. The help book consists of tab pages for the first session, second session, joint session and fourth session. According to what is happening in the life of the client, worksheets are added, which are used during and outside the session to support the client. The help book also contains information and psychoeducation for the client about the consequences of sexual abuse. Information about issues such as giving a police statement, medical tests and so on can be added, if applicable.

The help book also contains space for the client to draw their experiences and for the parents/carers, relatives and professional caregivers to do the same; preferably together with the client. The help book is for the client themselves and they bring it to the SOS sessions. Due to the fact that others also write in it, it also acts as a form of communication between all people involved.

It is recommended to use the help book at a fixed time. There are various reasons for this: on the one hand, this makes it easier to transfer that which has been learnt into real life; on the other hand, this provides a feeling of safety and trust that the victim is appreciated as a person. The caregivers need to be aware of the contents of the help book, so that they can refer to it, if and when necessary, according to the daily circumstances.

# General information and psychoeducation exercises

## Exercise: What has happened?

Draw here what has happened.

# Information sheet: Where does that strange feeling come from?

Most people who have experienced something bad have many different thoughts and feelings afterwards. Some people get a stomach ache, others can't sleep well or might feel restless, nervous or angry. Many people don't want to talk or think about the bad experience, but do, however, keep thinking about it.

Post-traumatic stress disorder (abbreviated as PTSD) is a collective name for the symptoms which you can suffer when you have had a bad experience. We have made a list of these after-effects. It is a long list of things which you *could* suffer. That doesn't mean that you *have* to suffer them. Most people have a few of these symptoms – which of them you experience varies per person. This is because everyone is different.

## Post-traumatic stress symptoms

*Feeling strange in your head*

- You find it difficult to concentrate.
- You are forgetful.
- You have a headache and don't know why.
- You are confused.
- You don't feel like doing anything.
- You don't enjoy things you used to enjoy.

*Feeling bad in your body*

- You feel tense.
- You are easily startled.
- You feel restless.
- You get angry quickly.
- You get scared quickly.
- You feel numb.

*You feel empty inside*

- You have a stomach ache or feel sick, and you don't know why.
- Your muscles hurt.

*Problems with sleeping*

- You find it difficult to get to sleep.
- You have nightmares or frightening dreams.
- You wake up quickly or very early.

*Thinking about it all the time*

- You have to keep thinking about what has happened, even if you don't want to.
- You see, hear or smell things, which make you think about what has happened.
- You sometimes suddenly see images or a film in your head of the bad thing you have experienced.

*Not daring to do things anymore*

- You do your best to avoid things which remind you of the bad experience. 'Avoid' means that you do your best not to come into contact with something.
- Things which you used to dare to do, you don't dare to do anymore.

If you have one or more of these symptoms, you will know where they come from. Usually these symptoms stop after a few weeks or months. If that isn't the case, and the symptoms worsen, then you must tell your parents, caregiver, doctor or someone else whom you trust and who can help you.[1]

1 Berlo, W. van, *et al.* (2011) *Beperkt weerbaareen onderzoek naar seksueel geweld bij mensen met een lichamelijke, zintuiglijke of verstandelijke beperking.* Utrecht: Rutgers WPF/Movisie.

# Information sheet: Post-traumatic stress symptoms

If you experience something bad, something happens in your body. This happens to everyone! Think about what happens if something shocks you… Your heart starts beating faster, your muscles tense, you begin to sweat or to shake, sometimes you are frightened or you get a headache or stomach ache. Your body sounds the alarm. When the bad situation has passed, you relax again, your heart starts beating normally and you calm down. Everything goes back to how it was before the bad situation started.

But sometimes the physical body keeps sounding the alarm, even after the incident has passed. The body stays tense and doesn't calm down. This means that you feel things such as fear, stomach ache, difficulty with sleeping or concentrating or becoming angry for no apparent reason. We use a difficult word for this: PTSD. That stands for: post-traumatic stress disorder.

*'Post'* means *'after'.*

*'Traumatic'* means *'horrible incident'.*

*'Stress'* means *'tension which doesn't go away'.*

You can suffer three things:

1. *Re-living experiences:* these are painful reminders of the horrible incident:
    - You keep having to think about the incident.
    - The horrible incident won't leave your head.
    - You see the horrible incident as a sort of film in your mind.
2. *Avoidance:* this means that you try not to come into contact with anything which will remind you of the horrible incident:
    - You try not to think about the horrible incident.
    - You would rather not talk about the horrible incident.
    - You avoid places or people.
    - You avoid situations which remind you of the horrible situation.

3. *Hyper-arousal:* this is a long word for all sorts of symptoms, such as:
   - Sleeping problems.
   - Getting angry quickly, sometimes about nothing.
   - Being irritable.
   - Not being able to concentrate at school.

## Worksheet: What is bothering you?

Sometimes people who have had a bad experience...

- have a stomach ache
- have bad dreams or nightmares
- think that friends know what has happened
- think that no one will like them
- don't enjoy things which they used to enjoy anymore
- don't want to think about the horrible incident, but can't stop thinking about it
- have sleeping problems
- think that they've done something bad
- don't do things they used to do anymore
- are scared to tell someone what has happened
- are scared that they will be punished if they tell someone what has happened
- have heard that something bad will happen to them if they tell anyone about what has happened
- believe that their body is dirty or ugly
- have problems with eating
- find it difficult to pay attention
- have problems at school
- are scared of danger
- are worried about what can happen.

### Important!

If you have experiences something horrible, it doesn't necessarily mean that you will have all of these symptoms. Maybe you are suffering symptoms which are not shown here. Everyone is different and has different symptoms. Make a list of things which are bothering you using the table below. Think about what could help you if it is bothering you.[1]

**List of symptoms**

| Symptom | Bothers you | Doesn't bother you | What helps? |
|---|---|---|---|
| Feeling strange in your head | | | |
| Feeling bad in your body | | | |
| Sleeping strangely | | | |
| Not daring to do things anymore | | | |
| Keep thinking about it | | | |
| | | | |
| | | | |
| | | | |

1 Gebruikgemaakt van: Plomp, F. *et al.* (2011) Conceptversie werkboek TFCGT kinderen en jongeren. Hengelo: Ambiq.

## Worksheet: How do I tell others about it?

It is important to talk about what has happened. This might be difficult, but it does help. This doesn't mean that you should talk to everyone about it. Let's make lists of the people you do and do not want to talk to. We will also think about how you can tell others about it. Maybe we will think together about what you can say yourself, but maybe we will think about what could help you or who could do that for you.

**I want to talk about it with...**

| Name | What am I going to say? |
|---|---|
| | |
| | |
| | |
| | |
| | |
| | |

**I don't want to talk about it with...**

| Name | What am I going to say if he or she asks about it or starts talking about it? |
|---|---|
| | |
| | |
| | |
| | |
| | |
| | |

## Worksheet: How have people reacted?

We have talked about how good and important it is to talk about what has happened with some people. Let's see how this went. We will also see how it went with people who you didn't want to talk with about it.

**I wanted to talk about it with...**

| Name | How did it go? | How did they react? |
|---|---|---|
| | | |
| | | |
| | | |
| | | |
| | | |
| | | |

**I didn't want to talk about it with...**

| Name | How did it go? |
|---|---|
| | |
| | |
| | |
| | |
| | |
| | |

## Safety exercises

### Worksheet: Who can I call?

People who have experienced something horrible often don't feel safe anymore.

To help you feel safe again, it helps to have a plan. Write on the drawing of the mobile phone who you can call for help, what their telephone number is and what you can say to them! Put it somewhere where you can find it easily, so that you can always look at it when you need to. Maybe it is also handy to put these numbers into your telephone.

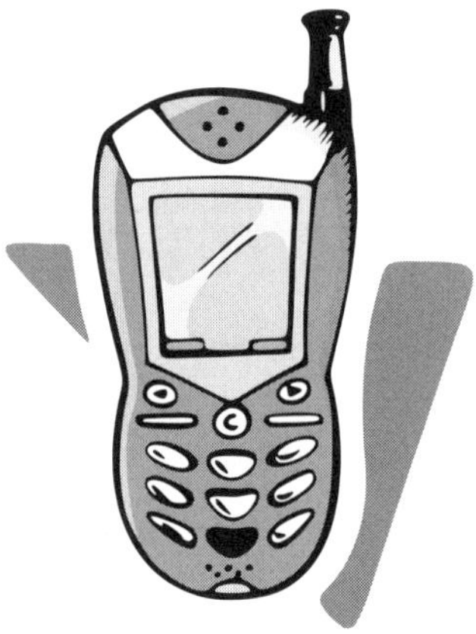

### I'm calling to say that...

- If something happens which makes me feel unsafe, then I will call ____________________ and then I'll say:

  ______________________________________________________________

  ______________________________________________________________

  ______________________________________________________________

  ______________________________________________________________

## Worksheet: Safety agreements

To be safe, and to feel safe, it is important to make agreements with people who can help you. Agreements have already been made to make sure that you are safe. We are going to write these agreements down together. Maybe you need to make other agreements, so that you will really feel safe. We will write these down as well. We will also see how we can make sure that you will get what you need!

**Agreements about safety**

| Which safety agreements have been made? | What do I still need to be able to feel safe? | How can we make sure this will happen? |
|---|---|---|
| | | |
| | | |
| | | |

# Worksheet: What was fine and good?

If you have experienced something bad, it is also very important to pay attention to the things which did go well, and to the things which you like and enjoy doing. It is important that you do these things, even if you really don't feel like doing them at first.

**Nice things**

| Nice things | What and with who? | How did I feel? |
|---|---|---|
| Being with people I trust | | |
| Doing fun things | | |
| Going to work or school | | |
| Looking after myself well | | |
| Something else which is important for me: | | |
| Something else which is important for me: | | |
| Something else which is important for me: | | |

# Worries exercises

## Worksheet: How am I doing?

On this page you can show how you are doing. Put a cross on the line. The nearer the cross is to the smiling face, the better it is going. Nearer the sad face means that it's not going so well.

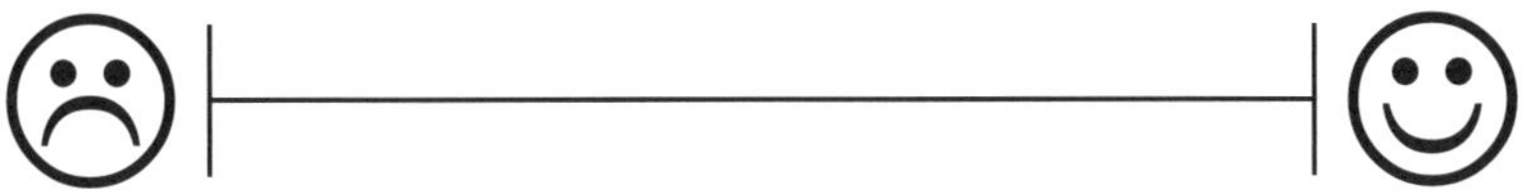

*How am I doing?*

## Worksheet: My worries are as big as...

Show how big you problems and worries are on this page. Are they like a mouse, like a tortoise or as big as an elephant? Write next to the relevant pictures which worries you have and what they are about.

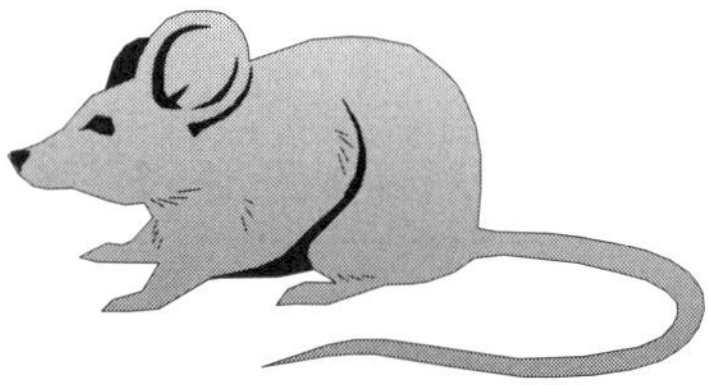

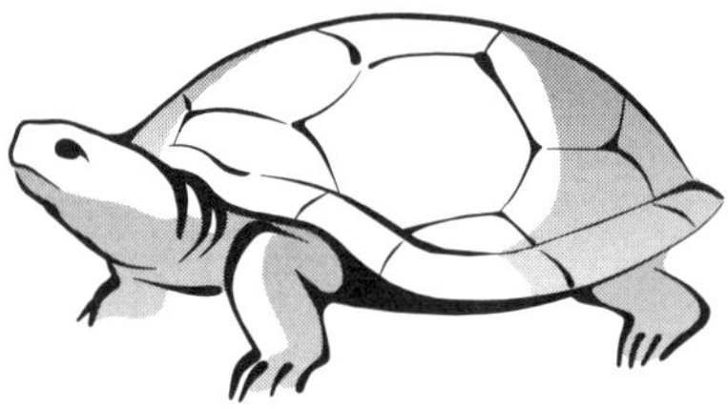

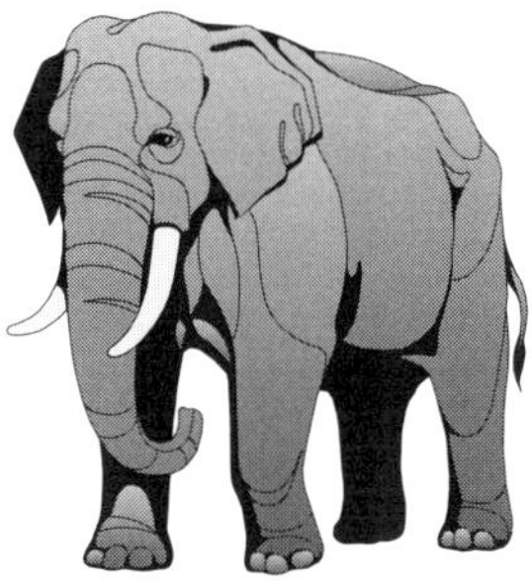

# Hurt exercises

## Worksheet: Your own tool box

If you have experienced horrible things, you can have awful feelings. That is normal. You can feel sad and terrible. But you can also *do* things to make you feel better; we're going to talk about that.

We're going to think and write down what you can do to feel better. We'll put these ideas in your own tool box. It is handy to have a box with tools, which can make you feel better. Then you can use them to feel better.

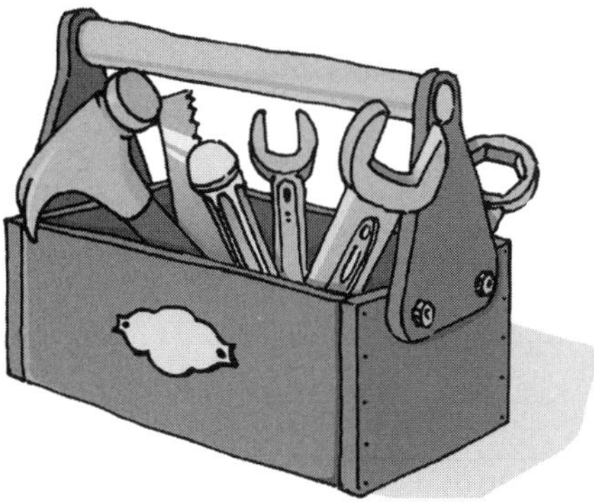

*Tool box*

Which things can you do to feel less awful?

______________________________

______________________________

______________________________

______________________________

______________________________

______________________________

## Worksheet: What can you *say* to yourself?

It is normal that people who have experienced something horrible will have awful feelings. You can deal with these feelings in all sorts of ways. You can *say* things to yourself to make yourself feel better; we're going to talk about that now.[1]

Here is a list of sentences which can help you. Say them aloud to yourself!

- What happened is not my fault!
- I'm not the only one. There are more people who have experienced this!
- People love me!
- I love myself!
- I deserve to feel well!
- I'm going to take good care of myself!

Think of some more things which you can say to yourself to make yourself feel better. Write them down here:

______________________________

______________________________

______________________________

______________________________

______________________________

______________________________

Which sentence do you like to hear the best?

______________________________

______________________________

______________________________

______________________________

______________________________

______________________________

1 Berlo *et al.* 2011.

# Fear exercises

## Worksheet: Important post

Think of a message from someone who is important to you, who could help you when you're scared. Write or draw the message in the envelope.

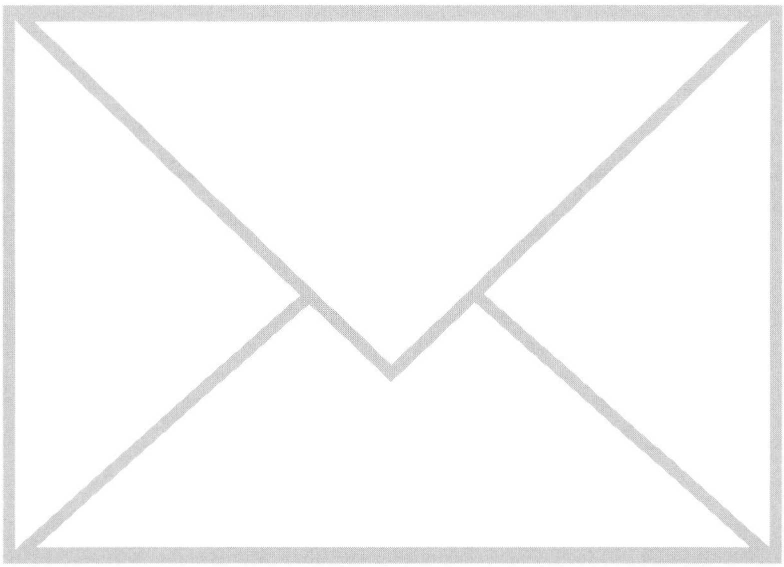

## Worksheet: My mask

If you are scared, you want to hide behind something and put on a mask. In that way, no one can see you and you are hidden away from the people or things which you are scared of. Today we are going to make a mask for you, just the way you want it to be, to hide behind if you are scared. When the mask is finished I will tell you: *'It would be nice to put this mask on when you are scared! But because you can't walk around with a mask on, we are going to think of other things to do if you are scared. What could help you to feel less scared?'*

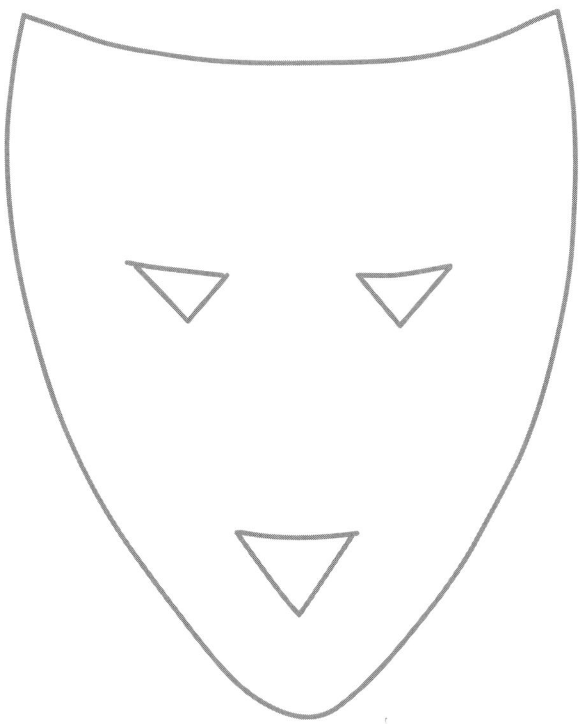

# Exercise: Fear, and then?

Everyone is scared sometimes. People who have experienced horrible things often feel more frightened. That is normal if you have experienced something bad.

Write down when you are scared and what you can do so that you won't be scared anymore.

**Actions for fear**

| | **When are you scared?** | **What can you do so that you're not scared anymore?** |
|---|---|---|
| 1 | | |
| 2 | | |
| 3 | | |
| 4 | | |
| 5 | | |
| 6 | | |
| 7 | | |

# Worksheet: Sleep-well plan

People who have experienced bad things often have problems sleeping. They are scared in the dark or have nightmares. Sometimes people are scared to go to sleep because they have such bad dreams.

In the sleep-well plan, you'll find things which will help you sleep better; tick the checklist and see what helps you sleep better.

**Sleep-well plan checklist**

| | Tick box |
|---|---|
| Look around in your bedroom to see if there are things, noises or scents which make you think about the horrible incident. Is there anything? Take these things away or put them in a different place. | |
| Make sure that you've got nice nightwear. | |
| Don't watch scary TV programmes before you go to sleep. | |
| Hang a card or a drawing on the wall with the text 'I'm safe now'. | |
| Put a nightlight on. | |
| Choose a fixed time to go to sleep and to get up in the morning. | |
| Make sure that you always do the same things before you go to bed, for example having a shower or reading a book. | |
| Don't sleep in the daytime. | |
| Make sure that it is not too warm in your bedroom. | |
| Make sure that you get enough exercise every day, so that you are actually tired when you go to bed. | |

## Exercise: Good night!

People who have experienced bad things have difficulty sleeping, others find it hard to calm down. Does this ever happen to you? If this is the case then you can do the following exercise at home. You can ask someone to read it to you if you want to calm down, or before you go to sleep, for example.

Lie down or sit in a nice place. A place which is peaceful and cosy (on the bed or sofa, for example). Breathe in slowly and breathe out even more slowly. Close your eyes. Imagine that you are floating on a soft cloud. You feel really safe on the cloud. Your whole body feels relaxed and heavy.

- Feel your feet. Your feet feel very relaxed. Your feet feel so heavy that it is difficult to lift them up.
- Feel your legs. Your legs feel really relaxed. Your legs are lying comfortably in the cloud.

It is a nice, warm and relaxed feeling. The feeling slowly travels up through your body: in your feet, in your legs.

- Feel your belly. Your belly feels very calm and full of warmth.
- Feel your chest. Your chest moves up and down slowly when you breathe. That feels calm and relaxing.
- Feel your neck and shoulders. They feel calm and heavy. Feel how your shoulders and your neck touch the clouds. You comfortably sink down a little into the cloud.
- Feel your head. Feel how relaxed your head is. Your head feels warm and heavy. Your head and face are relaxed. Your mouth and eyes feel nice and relaxed.
- Let your thoughts come and go, without worrying about them.

Everything is OK. You feel calm and good.

# Anger exercises

## Worksheet: The animal I look like the most when I'm angry is a...

Lots of people who experience bad things are angry, very angry. When we're angry we sometimes don't act like ourselves anymore. Then we say or do things, which we would not otherwise do. In the box below, draw the animal which you look like the most when you're angry.

How can you see that this animal is angry?

______________________________

How can someone else see that you are angry?

______________________________

What happens in your body when you are angry?

______________________________

# Exercise: Being angry in a good way

Many people who have experienced bad things feel angry. That is normal. You are allowed to feel angry about what has happened to you! It is OK to be angry. It is not OK if this makes you hurt yourself or others. It is important to find safe ways to be angry.

Safe ways to be angry:

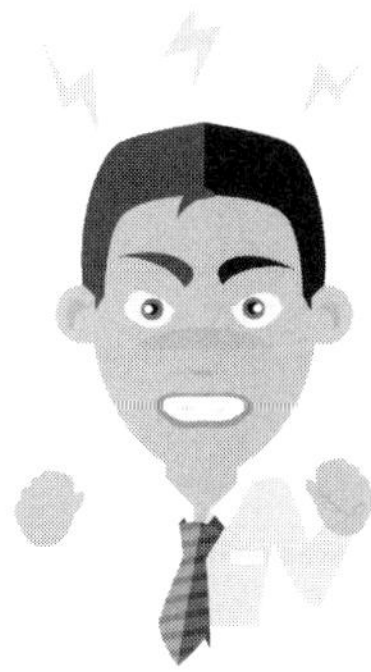

- hitting a cushion
- punching a punching bag
- going running
- screaming (out loud or in your head)
- kneading a stress ball
- throwing a (stress) ball hard against the wall
- tearing up paper
- scratching on paper
- talking about your anger with someone you trust or with your caregiver.

It is normal that you are angry. That's allowed. We do have to make sure that it is not going to bother you. That's why it's important that we think about a good way of being angry, without harming yourself or others. Write down your healthy ways to be angry.

## Exercise: Writing a letter

Write a letter about how angry you are.

In which way are you angry? Write underneath how you can be angry in a safe way (without hurting yourself or anyone else).

You could send the letter, but you don't have to.

## Exercise: Steam is coming out of my ears!

Many people who have experienced horrible things feel angry. This is normal. You are allowed to feel angry about what has happened to you!

We're going to draw what your face looks like when you're angry. Draw or write in the steam clouds, which are coming out of your ears, what you are very angry about.

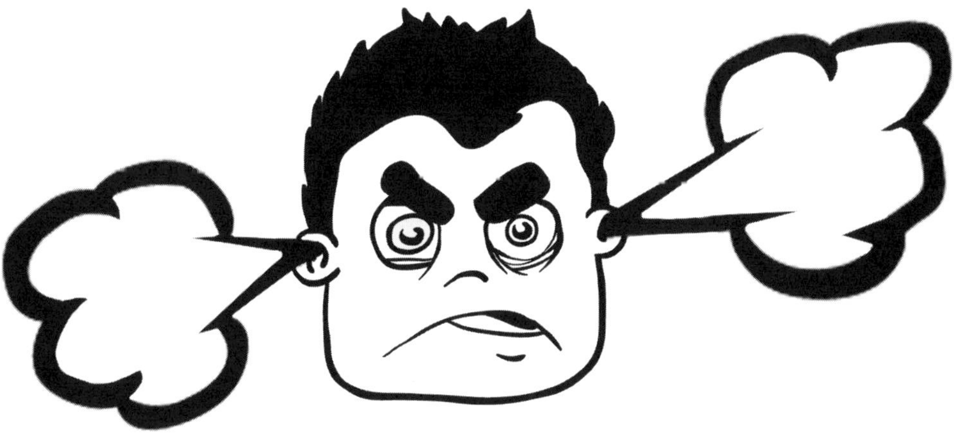

# Relaxation exercises

## Exercise: Blowing bubbles

Use a bubble-blowing container filled with soapy liquid. You can buy all sorts of these; big and small, made for girls or boys. Choose one which suits the client or adapt it to suit the client. It can do no harm to practise using it yourself beforehand.

Tell the client that it is important to do a relaxation exercise when you are feeling stressed. This helps you to calm down and feel better. It helps to breathe in and out deeply. One way to learn this is by blowing bubbles. Ask if the client has ever done this and how they found it. Tell them that you didn't know if you could do it yourself and that you have tried doing it a bit already.

Get the bubble-blowing container and ask the client to watch you when you blow bubbles. Ask the client to pay attention to your breath.

You take an exaggerated deep breath: 1-2-3, and when you blow out through the bubble blower you do that again slowly: 1-2-3. Repeat this a few times. Ask what the client sees and if they can copy this way of breathing. Practise this way of breathing with the client, during which you slowly count. 'Breathe in: 1-2-3...and breathe out again: 1-2-3.'

If the client can do that, get the bubble blower and let the client try doing it with the bubble blower.

Practise together with the client and give compliments about how it's going!

Add the worksheet to the help book and give the client the bubble blower to take home with them. Teach the caregivers to help the client to do this exercise and use the right breathing.

# Exercise: Colour

Find colouring pictures or mandalas which suit the client's personal interests.

Make sure you have got colouring pencils or pens.

Use two colouring pictures: one for yourself and one for the client. Ask the client to take their time colouring in the picture. Tell the client to concentrate on the point of the pencil or pen and ask them to colour in the picture slowly and as well as possible.

Tell the client that this is a good way to calm down. Colouring slowly and with concentration helps to relax. Act as a role model and colour as much as possible alongside the client.

Practise with the client and pay them compliments!

Add the worksheet to the help book and give it to the client to take home with them. Add a number of colouring pictures or mandalas. Teach the caregivers how they can help the client use this exercise for relaxation purposes.

## Exercise: Spaghetti arms

Tell the client that when you feel tense, it is important to do a relaxation exercise. This relaxes you and helps you to feel better. Tell them that there are many different ways to relax. One of these is to pay attention to how tense your arms and shoulders feel when you're stressed, or very angry, and to learn to let go of this feeling.

Put your chair opposite the client's chair. Say: 'We're going to try doing this now. Sit down comfortably on your chair.' Show the client how you do this.

Ask the client to clench their fists as hard as possible and slowly count to three. Then ask the client to relax their fists and arms and to shake them to release the tension. Count 1-2-3. Repeat a few times. The last time you say:

*'This time we're going to count to ten when you relax your fists and arms. I want you to relax your arms, so that they feel like they were made of spaghetti. Let's begin.'*

After you have done this, ask the client what they have noticed about their arms and how it felt. If the client says that they didn't feel anything, repeat the exercise again and give the instructions: *'Pay attention to your neck and arms. Are they tense and tight when you clench your fists?'*

When the client relaxes their muscles, ask: *'And now? How can we make them into spaghetti?'*

Act as a role model during the exercise and do as much as possible together. Practise with the client and pay them compliments!

Add the worksheet to the help book and give this to the client. Teach the caregivers to help the client use this exercise.

## Exercise: Relax!

When people experience bad things, their body sometimes stays in a state of alarm, even when the bad experience has passed. Your body stays in a state of tension, which causes all kinds of symptoms (stomach ache, fear, sleeping problems, getting angry for no apparent reason). It is important that you learn how you can *relax* your body.

Relaxation is about feeling calm and peaceful. You feel better when you are relaxed. But...how do you do that, relax? With this exercise for tensing and relaxing muscles, for example:

Sit down quietly on your chair with your arms on your legs and your feet on the ground. Close your eyes. Imagine that you have got a ball of clay in your hand. Squeeze as tightly as you can in the ball of clay. When you squeeze, feel how tense the muscles of your hand and arm are. Count to five and let the ball of clay fall out of your hands. Let your hands hang loosely. Feel the difference in the muscles of your hand and arm, now that they are relaxed. Say to yourself: 'My hand is relaxed'. Now do the same with your other hand.

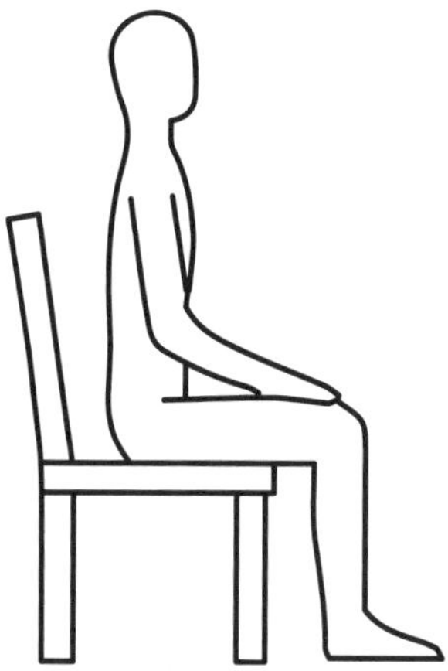

*Sit down quietly on a chair*

You can do this exercise with different parts of your body: hands, arms, feet, legs, belly, back, chest, shoulders, face. You can do this with the different body parts, one at a time, or all at the same time. What do you want to do?[1]

1 Berlo *et al.* 2011.

## Exercise: Belly breathing

When you feel bad, you sometimes forget to breathe! Or you breathe quickly and shortly, just like a dog panting. You can do the belly breathing to relax.

When you breathe in deeply and then out even more slowly, you breathe through your belly. When you breathe in you count to five, when you breathe out, you count to six (and further, if possible!).

When you breathe in, your belly gets bigger, when you breathe out, it gets smaller again. You can compare this to a balloon. When a balloon is blown up, it gets bigger. When the air is let out of the balloon, it shrinks. The balloon does the same thing as your belly.

Use a balloon to show how big your belly appears when you breathe in and how it shrinks when you breathe out. You blow the balloon up when you breathe in and let the air out slowly when you breathe out. Act as a role model during the exercise and do as much as possible together with the client.

Practise with the client and pay them compliments!

Ask the client to teach the belly breathing to someone who looks after them (parents, educators or caregivers). Let the client practise at least once a day.

Add the worksheet to the help book and give it to the client to take home with them. Teach the caregivers to help the client to do this exercise.

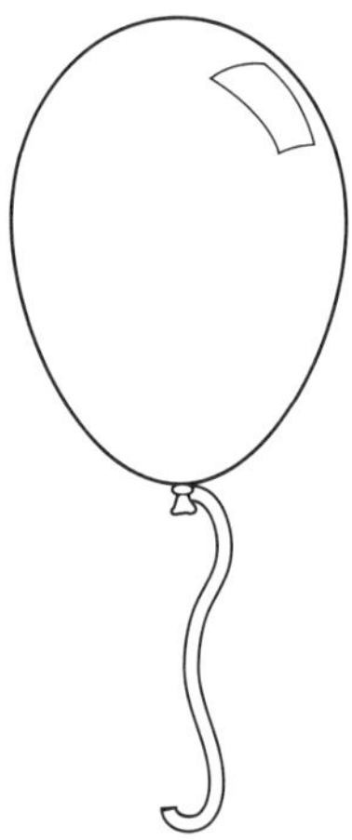

*Belly breathing is like a balloon*

# Survival exercises

## Exercise: Sunshine after rain

When it rains, it doesn't keep raining for ever, does it? Even if it sometimes feels like it does, there always comes a day when the sun shines again.

Worries are not there forever either. With some problems and worries it seems as if you can't do anything to lessen them or to stop them. Nothing seems to help. Then it is just like with the rain. We can't stop that either. But it always stops raining sometime! Yes, it really does! And when it rains, we can always think of something to do until the rain stops again. Of course we can! We don't just sit and wait.

### What helps?

What can we do to make your life more enjoyable until your problems (your rain) are over?

1. ______________________________
2. ______________________________
3. ______________________________
4. ______________________________

## Exercise: Four-leaf clover

Here you can see a four-leaf clover. Write or draw on every leaf a message for someone who is important to you. Write down which fun things you would like to do with that person.

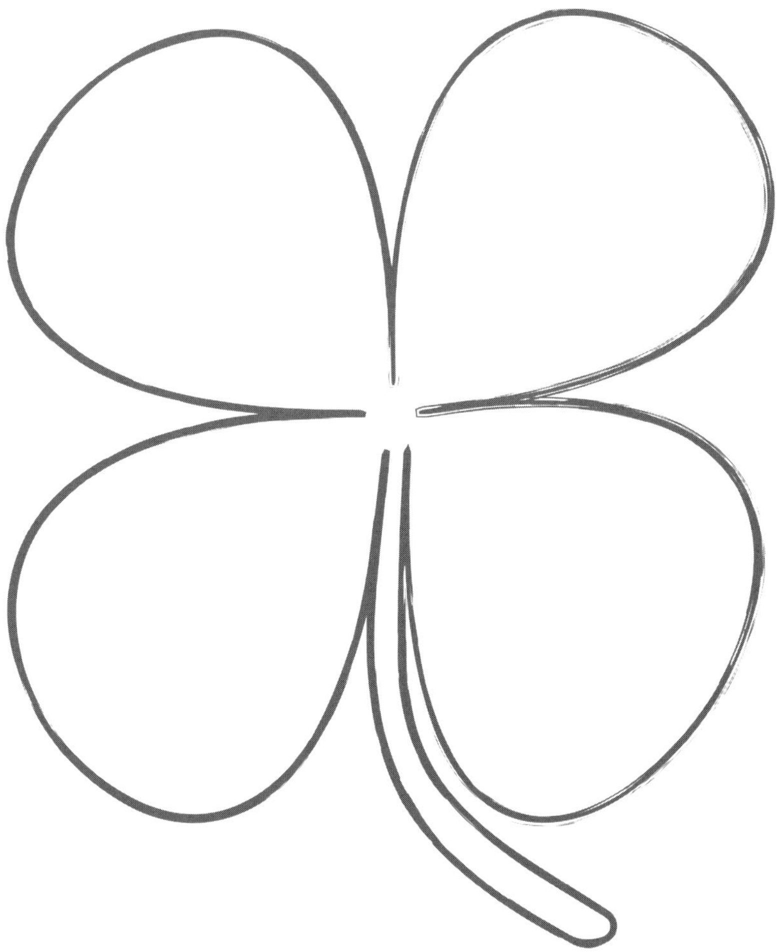

## Exercise: Looking into the future

Imagine that you can look into the future. How do you see yourself and your life in 10 or 20 years' time? Write in the mirror how you see your future.

# Exercise: Wishing well

Here you seen a wishing well? When people throw a coin into the well, they can make a wish. You have got three coins to throw into the well. What do you wish?

My three wishes:

1. ______________________________
2. ______________________________
3. ______________________________

## Exercise: Together we are strong – the plaster

The 'Together we are strong' exercise is done in the third, joint session of the SOS programme. You'll need a strong piece of paper or thin cardboard for this, on which the professional has drawn a big plaster.

You introduce the exercise and explain, in a way which is suited to the level of the client, that abuse hurts.

*'It is not exactly the same as having a wound on your body, but it is the same sort of thing. When you have a wound on your body, you stick a plaster on it. That helps to let it heal more quickly. The plaster keeps the dirt out and protects the wound, also if you bump into something. If your feelings have been wounded (or your heart or your spirit or whatever you would like to call it) then you can't stick a real plaster on it. But what we can do is make a beautiful plaster for the wound together. Then we can imagine that we are sticking it over the pain in your heart. You can hang this plaster up in your (bed) room. You can look at it whenever you feel bad. Then you'll remember that we are all supporting and helping you and that we want to give you the plaster so that you'll feel less pain. We're going to make the plaster as beautiful as possible together and decorate it so that it will really suit you!'*

Then everyone joins in decorating the plaster. The plaster should be drawn large enough for everyone to be able to work on it at the same time. During the process, the client is asked what they think of it: if they like the colours, the pictures and so on. While working, those present make positive statements about the characteristics of the client. The plaster is finished when it has been coloured in completely and the client is happy with it. When it is finished, tell the client again why the plaster has been made. It is also possible to hang the plaster up together in the room afterwards.

# Exercise: Together we are strong – the message

The 'Together we are strong' exercise is done in the third, joint session of the SOS programme. For this exercise a large piece of paper is needed and a mobile telephone (or a computer with a large screen). You introduce the exercise and explain that it is very important after sexual abuse that you know that everyone is there to help you.

*'You're not alone. People who have experienced horrible things sometimes forget that. And they forget to look for help when they are feeling bad. To help remind you to do that, we're going to think of a few messages which can help. Everyone will think of one line to help him/her and we will make a beautiful story together. We'll begin by all writing a few sentences and reading them to you. You can say if the sentence should be in the story or not.'*

A variation on this exercise is writing song lyrics about receiving help. When the story is finished, it is written on a separate piece of paper and decorated, if required. Then a photo can be made on the client's mobile phone, so that the story can go everywhere with them.

## Exercise: Together we are strong – the song

The 'Together we are strong' – exercise is done in the third joint session of the SOS programme. For this exercise, a karaoke set is required, recording equipment and people involved who enjoy music and singing. It is important to find this out beforehand.

You introduce the exercise and explain that making a song for, and together with, the client can help in difficult times, when everyone isn't together. A simple song is chosen. A text is made together, focusing on how the future is going to get better. As a professional, make sure that the song isn't about bad things, but is instead supportive and positive. It is possible to prepare this yourself in advance.

## Chapter 7

# HELP BOOK FOR PEOPLE WITH A SEVERE INTELLECTUAL DISABILITY

## Introduction

People with a severe intellectual disability who have suffered sexual abuse are often not able to make sense of what has happened to them. When these people suffer sexual abuse and the perpetrator is a significant other, their ability to trust is damaged. The client experiences that the person whom they trust is also the one who hurts them. The need for protection, which these clients display in both physical and emotional terms, becomes threatening and unsafe; creating an unsolvable problem. The client can develop a tendency to avoid emotional contact and to become withdrawn.

After sexual abuse, the client will become confused about physical contact. They will have the tendency to repeat what has happened to them in their own behaviour and in this way can be labelled as sexually attention seeking or provocative. People with a severe intellectual disability often cannot express with language what has happened to them. Communication takes place through behaviour.

For this group of people, support after sexual abuse focuses primarily on restoring safety and trust in the people surrounding them, on whom the client depends. The client must be helped in calming the stress response system, the neurological regulatory system that is disrupted after a traumatic experience and quickly goes into overdrive. It is necessary that clients with a severe intellectual disability are able to experience a feeling of safety and predictability in actions, language and at a sensory level, in the contact with their caregivers and parents.

## 7.1 People with a severe intellectual disability

The target group of people with a severe intellectual disability is extremely diverse. A severe intellectual disability is generally indicated when the developmental level of the client is below three years old.

When you consider the vast differences in development of people in the first three years of their lives – from a helpless baby to a headstrong and adventurous toddler – it becomes clear that it is impossible to generalise. Additional problems are often also present, which determine the way in which people with a severe intellectual disability function. The type and severity of disabilities and disorders, combined with the positive factors of development, are therefore diverse.

There are differences in the way in which people respond to sensory information from the environment, for example, and how they demonstrate this. Some clients are extremely open to the world around them. Sensory information seems to just stream in. Other clients have a closed character. These people often don't seem to register sensory information. An open or closed character is often connected to a hyper or hypo sensitivity of the senses.[1] Individual attention and a great amount of sensitivity are essential in building a relationship and in carrying out activities with these people.

This emphasises the fact that the professional conducting the SOS programme needs to be aware of the lifestory of the individual person with a severe intellectual disability, while also considering the positive factors of development (see Section 5.2.2). For this reason, it is of great importance to involve parents and/or family in the programme, in order to be able to consider essential personal information.

The complexity of the disability is determined by the way in which the cognitive and additional disorders interfere with, influence and reinforce each other.

A theoretical distinction can be made between cognitive, social and emotional aspects regarding the psychosocial development of people with a severe intellectual disability. The lower the developmental level, the harder it is to distinguish between the different aspects.

### 7.1.1 Cognitive aspect

The thought processes of a person with a low developmental level of functioning/severe intellectual disability show many weaknesses. There is no awareness of cause and effect in their minds and it is difficult for them to think about things or people who are not actually present in the current situation. Additionally, their thought processes are strongly egocentric: for these clients it is impossible to empathise with others. These people demonstrate limited understanding of the world around them.

Most people with a severe intellectual disability use little to no language as a means of communication. It is impossible for them to do or show something in actions which they have not themselves experienced or seen.

### 7.1.2 Social aspect

With regard to the social aspect, these clients are able to interact with others, but are not, however, able to show reciprocal behaviour. Empathising with another person is impossible at this developmental level. There is a great dependency on the carer, who forms a bridge to the rest of the world. Some clients function at the imitation stage of development.

### 7.1.3 Emotional aspect

From an emotional perspective there is a great dependency on the carer. They need to do things together, to participate and to imitate. They generally have little to no impulse control and can be overwhelmed by their emotions. Emotions such as happiness, anger, sadness and fear have usually been developed. Anger can be displayed, directed at significant others.

Considering the development of personal character, it can be said that the ego is fragile and dependent.

## 7.2 Sexual abuse and people with a severe intellectual disability

It was long thought that people with a severe intellectual disability who have suffered sexual abuse were immune to the consequences. People thought that they would quickly forget such incidents and would continue to live in the 'here and now'. The assumption was that the suffering of these people would be less, due to the fact that they do not understand the meaning of what has happened to them. It is, however, becoming increasingly clear that serious incidents which are not cognitively understood do actually cause physical memories which can consciously or subconsciously affect people for years afterwards.

It is often still thought that people with a low developmental level of functioning suffer less, due to the fact that they cannot communicate about what is troubling them. Unfortunately, the reality is different. People with a severe intellectual disability often do experience problems as a consequence of abuse and mistreatment and they also actually communicate these problems. However, this is not usually expressed in words, but in behavioural signs.

### 7.2.1 Physical contact

People with a severe intellectual disability are often almost completely dependent on their surroundings. This is the case with nearly all daily actions, depending on the person and their level of development. In order to exercise influence on their surroundings, people with a severe intellectual disability need to experience relationships with other people who understand and fulfil their needs. Due to the developmental phase in which people with a severe intellectual disability function, a great deal of physical contact is necessary in order to combat feelings of helplessness. People are fed and changed and so on. Close contact and trusted rhythms help people with a severe intellectual disability to feel safe in contact with others and have enough trust to have an open approach to physical contact. Sexual abuse damages this basic feeling of safety and fades the already fragile sense of physical boundaries and autonomy. It takes away trust in the world around them, while at the same time people with a severe intellectual disability are constantly dependent on the people around them. This creates a constant sense of fear and insecurity, from which physical escape is impossible. Disengagement (dissociation) from the here and now is for this group the only way out of the situation.

See Chapter 4 for more about coping with trauma for people with an intellectual disability.

## 7.3 Core aspects in psychological support of people with a severe intellectual disability

One of the greatest challenges for the professional – and a requirement for conducting the programme – is to understand the way in which the client communicates. This is often not simple, because the lower the developmental level of people with a disability, the less able they are to communicate with spoken language. Most professionals have such little contact with individual clients that they do not have the opportunity to learn to read the signs themselves. In order to read the signs which people with a severe intellectual disability show, it is essential to work together with professional caregivers and/or parents, who know the person well and are alert to the signs. Due to the limited possibilities for communication and the limited behavioural repertoire of these people, the consequences of sexual abuse are often difficult to recognise. Each change in behaviour could signify an after-effect and deserves consideration as to whether or not it is related to the abuse. These changes could concern physical problems, developmental stagnation, apathetic behaviour, sudden eating problems, resistance to physical care or fixation on sexual organs.

The problems which people with a severe intellectual disability experience after abuse and mistreatment are generally comparable to the problems which young children (0–3 years) experience after abuse. Working with this target group requires patience, small steps and a low tempo, combined with much repetition.

### 7.3.1 Observation

Sandra Hewitt, psychologist and researcher in the US in the subject of young children and sexual abuse, has developed a short screening list for young children up to 36 months of age. This list has also proved helpful in working with children and adults with a severe intellectual disability.[2] Three main areas are described in this screening list, which act as guidelines for observations:

- change in emotions and behaviour regulation
- atypical sexual behaviour
- aversive situational reactions.

This screenings list is included in the help book (Section 7.4).

### 7.3.2 Calming sensory experiences

The SOS programme for people with a severe intellectual disability focuses primarily on restoring safety and trust in the people and the environment on which the client is dependent. The stress response system must be calmed. This neurological regulatory system is disrupted after a traumatic experience and quickly goes into overdrive (see Chapter 4). First, calming sensory experiences are provided as calming the 'arousal state' is the main priority. As long as this system remains in a state of defence, no other information can be registered, making recovery impossible.

The use of calming sensory experiences is necessary because the experience of abuse – partly due to the severe intellectual disability – is not remembered in language, but is predominantly recorded in a sensory way in the brain.[3, 4] For these clients, it is necessary that they experience safety and predictability, not only in language and actions of caregivers and parents, but also at a sensory level.

Alongside the exercises given in the help book, the information in the 'Sensory integration and Sherborne approach' can provide many additional ideas.[5]

## 7.4 The help book for the client with a severe intellectual disability

For people with a severe intellectual disability, the help book largely fulfils a guiding function for the significant people in their life. It functions as a tool for communication and reference. Before the sessions take place, the professional puts the help book together and adds to it at each session.

The practitioner can use a folder with various tab pages. The help book consists of the tab pages for the first session, second session, joint session and fourth session. The screenings list from Hewitt is added as a starting point and is read and filled in by those involved before each SOS session.

The exercises which are to be used in the session are added and a record is made of how the exercise went during the session. Additionally, after each session, a page is added which describes how, with whom and when the exercises will be included in the daily life of the client. There is also space on the page for a short report of how the exercises work.

The exercises are divided into themes (safety, worries, hurt, fear, anger, relaxation and survival) and can be chosen depending on the situation and what suits the client. Putting together the help book and the choice of the exercises depends on the individual circumstances of the client. There is not a fixed list of contents for the help book, as this would not do justice to the different situations which are encountered in real life.

In the previous chapter exercises are described which could also be of help to a number of clients with a severe intellectual disability (Section 6.3). If that is the case, then these worksheets are also added to the help book.

### *Sessions with the professional*

For this target group, we have also chosen to conduct four sessions in the presence of a professional, in order to structure the support provided. This gives the support a formal structure and fixed times, and co-operation between those involved is initiated.

As previously described, the sessions for these people should be adapted to the situation discussed together, also with regard to the length of the session and the meeting place. The roles and tasks during the session change depending on the developmental level of the client. The starting point is that the lower the client's level, the more the professional fulfils the role of coach during the sessions, and the more the caregiver or parent actually conducts the activities. Also, the lower the functional level of the client, the greater the importance that the exercises introduced during the sessions are also conducted daily or even more frequently between the sessions.

### *Two-part help book*

The help book for people with a severe intellectual disability consists of two parts. In the first part, general information is provided and practical lists can be found. The second part consists of suggestions for exercises in the areas of safety, worries, hurt, fear, anger, relaxation and survival.

It is of great importance that people with a severe intellectual disability experience routine and continuity, both during and outside the sessions. For people with severe intellectual disabilities, it is recommended that a physiotherapist is consulted about the best way in which exercises focusing on this theme can be conducted.

# General information and psychoeducation exercises

## Information sheet: Short screening list for sexual abuse of people with a severe intellectual disability

### Emotional dysregulation and behaviour dysregulation

Regression in acquired developmental skills:

- reduced awareness/apathy
- regression in toilet training
- loss of communication
- restlessness in movements or rigidity of movement
- increase in stereotypical behaviour
- strange new stereotypical behaviour
- often being unwell.

Increased fear of separation:

- cries on separation
- refuses to be separated from another person
- refuses to go to certain places.

Sleep disturbance:

- restlessness when going to bed
- difficulty falling asleep
- frequently waking up in the night
- frequent nightmares and fears
- reversal of day–night rhythm.

Disruption of emotions:

- sudden anger or aggression
- new fears
- socially withdrawn
- self-harm

- (hyper) vigilance
- startled reactions
- not wanting to be touched
- crying inconsolably.

## Abnormal sexual behaviour

- repeating sexual actions
- repeatedly doing things or doing things in a certain order (washing, putting things in and out of something)
- performing sexual actions with dolls
- repeating sounds or actions which are associated with sexual actions, for example rubbing sexual body parts against toys
- initiating sexual games with others
- putting things in the vagina or anus.

## Averse situational reactions

- talking about sexual actions or experiences
- increased and extra attention for sexually tinted things
- flashbacks
- former sexual behaviour returns
- new allegations
- constantly repeating sexual actions
- dreams/nightmares
- fears coming back when confronted with things which are related to the abuse.

## Behavioural signs which can relate to the type of abuse they have suffered

- *Violent or sudden abuse*: after-effects often begin with sudden fears, sleeping problems and unusual sexual behaviour. A feeling of fear or anxiety can be expressed in behaviour.
- *Slow build-up of abuse without violence:* clients show a keen interest in sexual games or objects. They can behave in a fearful way (sleep disorders, fear or anxiety). In addition there is sexualised behaviour, in which the client can also involve others.

## Form: Observations and experiences regarding the screening list per session

Session 1:

Session 2:

Session 3:

Session 4:

# Form: Agreements and experiences of conducting the exercises in the daily situation

Exercise: ______________________________

Conducted by: ______________________________

How did it go?

______________________________

______________________________

______________________________

______________________________

Exercise: ______________________________

Conducted by: ______________________________

How did it go?

______________________________

______________________________

______________________________

______________________________

Exercise: ______________________________

Conducted by: ______________________________

How did it go?

______________________________

______________________________

______________________________

______________________________

# Safety exercises

## Exercise: Restoring safety and making contact

*Lap exercises: rocking, singing and imitation games.* Due to the level of intensive physical contact, it is preferable for the parent to conduct these exercises.

Sit the client on your lap, with the client's back against the front of the adult. Sing songs while rocking back and forth. Hold the client's hand while doing so. This helps the client to experience the situation as being safe.

If the client is positioned the other way round on the adult's knees, then they can look at each other. Eye contact can be encouraged by clapping hands.

Tips per disability:

- If the client is partially sighted or blind, it helps to put some music on and to sing along to it.
- Make sure that other disturbing sounds (for example, from a TV, music or computer) are turned off; this will otherwise cause distraction.
- If the client is hard of hearing or deaf, provide visual sensory information. Go and sit in a multi-sensory stimulation room, for example. The client will then experience physical contact and will be calmed by the visual sensory information in the space. For some clients, bodily contact is enough on its own.

## Exercise: Colour

Ask the client to choose a colouring picture (for example, on www.kleurplaten.nl) and colour this in. Sit with them and also colour in a colouring picture. Colouring together creates a feeling of calm and togetherness.

# Worries exercises

## Exercise: How are you doing?

We want to know how you are doing and how things are going in your life. Put a cross on the line in the image below. The nearer the cross is to the laughing face, the better things are going. A cross nearer the sad face means that it's not going so well.

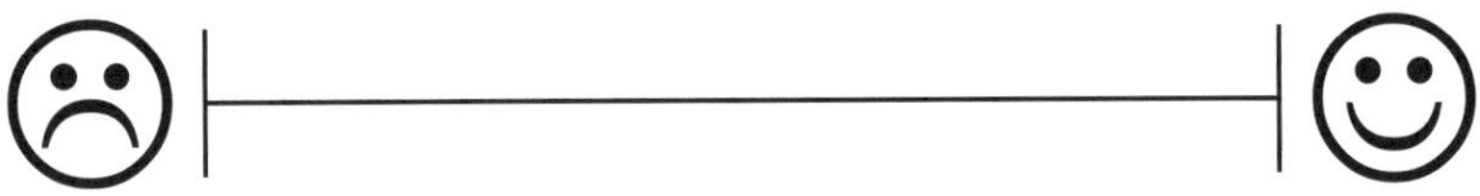

## Exercise: The elephant

Introduction:

*'Sometimes we worry about things a lot. Then it seems as if our worries are as big as an elephant! Look, we've got an elephant here. Make a drawing of your worries on the elephant.'*

You can also say that you yourself can write or draw things for the client and then ask the client to colour in the elephant further.

When the client is finished colouring, tell them:

*'I know that it is difficult to put what has happened out of your mind when your worries are as big as an elephant. But there are things that can help. Shall we think of what can help you to think about other things?'*

Think together with the client about what they can do (visiting people they trust, playing a game on the computer, doing jobs in the house and so on). Write these things down next to the elephant on the page.

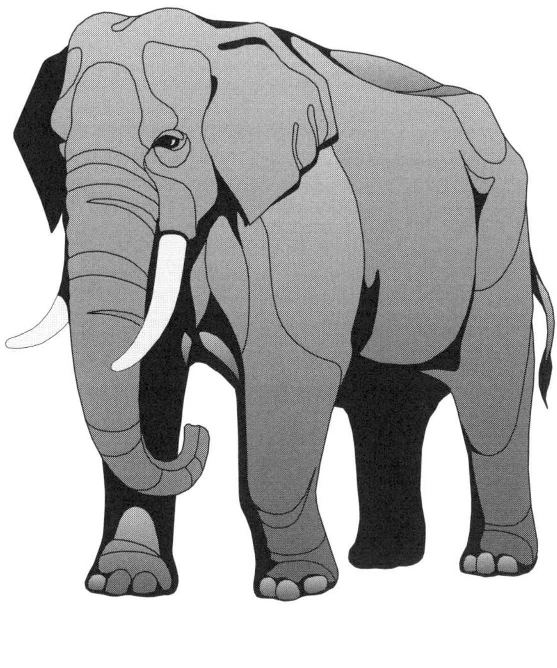

# Hurt exercise

## Exercise: Swinging

Swinging is an activity which helps people feel better. Swinging helps to calm disturbed parts of the brain. Swinging can be done in different ways: in a swinging chair, together or alone. It is also possible to swing in the playground on a normal swing, with hair blowing in the wind. It can also be done on a swing-boat.

Choose the form which suits the client best and suits the mood they are in. Swinging can, of course, also be accompanied by singing.

## Worksheet: Sleep-safe plan

Clients who have experienced bad things, often have sleeping problems. They are often scared of the dark or are troubled by nightmares. Sometimes they are scared of going to sleep because they have such bad dreams.

A number of things are mentioned which can help with sleeping better. Tick the checklist and see what is appropriate for the client to do. Add things to the list which suit the individual client.

**Safe sleep checklist**

| | **Check!** |
|---|---|
| Look around in the bedroom to see if there are things, noises or scents which remind the client of the bad incident. If so, take these things away or put them in a different place. | |
| Make sure that the client wears nice nightwear. | |
| Consider using a weighted blanket. | |
| Choose a fixed sleeping routine, in which reassurance is the main thing. | |
| Put a nightlight on. | |
| Make sure that someone is nearby when the client goes to sleep. | |
| | |
| | |
| | |
| | |

# Exercise: Look for the triggers

People who have experienced abuse often become scared of things which remind them of what has happened. If a situation such as this occurs, the body reacts with the reflex of fear. It is important for parents and caregivers to be alert to these triggers, recognise them and where possible prevent them. If prevention is not possible, it is important to help the client to get through the situation safely by providing reassurance.

The following list can be used to track down triggers, to see how the client reacts to them and to keep a record of what helps. Whether or not the reaction to the triggers stops after a few weeks can also be noted here. A number of suggestions are given, which may or may not be appropriate for the individual situation.

**Triggers for fear**

| Trigger | Reaction | What helps? |
|---|---|---|
| 1. Place where it happened | Rigidity, crying | Avoiding this place |
| 2. Changing time, walking to the place where the changing is done, when it is time to get changed... | Resistance, anger, walking away | |
| 3... | | |
| 4... | | |
| 5... | | |

# Anger exercises

## Exercise: Rubbish bin/tin can throwing game

For the exercise 'tin can throwing', a number of large metal rubbish bins or tin cans are needed, alongside a toilet roll and a bowl or bucket of water. A tower is made out of the 'cans'. The client makes wet paper balls, consisting of toilet roll and water, to throw with.

This exercise is introduced by saying:

*'The horrible thing which you experienced can make you angry and want to break things. That feeling is fine and it is all right. What we are going to do now will help you to let this feeling be there in a good way, without hurting anybody. You'll feel better afterwards. Shall we try to throw the bins over as hard as possible?'*

It is important to show the client how they can make a paper ball and to encourage them to throw as hard as possible and to join in yourself. The main aim is expressing strength, and experiencing the noise and sound of the wet paper balls.

Variation: if the client is angry with a certain person (the perpetrator), you can hang a large piece of paper on the inside of the door. Possibly together with others, the client draws the perpetrator on this piece of paper. The client throws the wet paper balls at the head of the perpetrator.

## Exercise: Tearing paper

For this exercise, a large pile of coloured tissue paper is needed and also a box, a piece of paper, emotions pictograms and glue. Together with others, the client tears the paper into pieces, making a sort of big confetti. The torn paper is thrown in a box or container. When it is finished, all the paper is thrown up in the air, creating a coloured rainstorm of paper.

This exercise is introduced by saying:

*'The horrible thing which you experienced can mean that you are angry and would like to break things. That feeling is fine and all right. What we are now going to do will help you to show this feeling in a good way without hurting anybody. You'll feel better afterwards. We are going to make confetti by tearing the paper up with all of our strength. Shall I show you how?'*

Begin by tearing the paper and help the client to start doing so as well.

*'When it is finished, we will have made a whole box full, which we will throw over our heads. We'll try to keep the pieces in the air for as long as possible.'*

Make a game out of it. When it is finished, say:

*'Now we need to take some deep breaths. Do you know what we'll do now? We'll choose a few beautiful pieces of paper and stick them on a piece of paper. Then we'll write down the word 'angry' (or stick the pictogram of angry on the page). Then we'll know that it is OK to be angry.'*

# Relaxation exercises

## Exercise: Bubble blowing

Blowing bubbles is a beautiful way to let the client with a lower level of development practise deep breathing. Deep breathing contributes to relaxation.

Make sure that you have a least two bubble blowers (depending on the number of participants) and begin blowing beautiful bubbles. Invite the client to do the same thing and possibly take turns blowing bubbles or blow them together at the same time. Breathing out can be practised between bubble blowing by holding a competition in 'blowing out for as long as possible'.

## Exercise: Hand and foot massage

Hand and foot massage provides relaxation. The senses are stimulated and the physical contact can strengthen the relationship between the parent/relative and caregiver. The client also experiences a sense of their own body.

Make sure that the room is warm, and that the hands are warm as well. It is possible to bath the client beforehand, so that they feel completely relaxed.

Due to the abuse, it is best to only massage the hands and/or feet and to carefully observe how the client experiences the massage. It is also fine to massage the client for a short time the first time in order to let them get used to the touch and the oil.

While massaging the client's hands, cover the rest of their body so that they stay warm.

Tips per disability:

- If the client is partially sighted or blind, it is important to name all actions which are done. In this way nothing unexpected happens.
- Possibly use oil with a strong, pleasant scent.

# Survival exercise

## Exercise: Together we are strong – music

For this exercise, musical instruments or a music system with loudspeakers are required.

The professional introduces the exercise beforehand to the parents/relatives and the care team and explains that sexual abuse causes victims to feel alone and isolated. It is especially important to the client to break through this feeling of isolation and to let them experience that we are standing strong together and that the client is part of a greater whole.

*'Because we can't do that with words, it is essential to let the client experience this. Music and singing is a good way of doing this. Let's think together which music we can use to express this feeling and how we can organise it.'*

Parents/relatives and care team members usually know which music the client prefers. It is a good idea to practise together once in the preparatory meeting.

On the day of the session, if a music system is used, all those involved sit together in a circle and hold each other's hands. In this way the client is part of the circle. The group can rock/move together while singing.

If musical instruments and music making is chosen, everyone stands around the client and the client is given a role in the music making.

A recording can be made of the music so that it can be played at other moments.

Chapter 8

# SUPPORT OF PARENTS OF VICTIMS OF SEXUAL ABUSE WITH AN INTELLECTUAL DISABILITY

## Introduction

The central topic in this chapter is the support for parents of children with an intellectual disability who are victims of sexual abuse.[1] Supporting the parents and relatives is an essential part of the SOS programme. This also applies when clients are not children themselves anymore and when the contact between parent and child is less intensive.

People with an intellectual disability are often very closely connected to their families, and their families to them, up into old age, even when this doesn't appear to be the case. This is partly due to the fact that the client often has to deal with many different professional caregivers; the family is then the only constant factor in the life of a person with a disability. It is also often the case that the family, due to the intellectual disability of their child, feels a high level of care and concern for their children for a longer period of time than most parents feel for children who grow up without a disability. Moreover, people with an intellectual disability, in comparison with others, are largely dependent on, and influenced by, their surroundings. This means that the reactions and coping strategies of those around them are a crucial factor in how the child copes with the situation.

The same after-effects and symptoms are often seen in parents and relatives as in the client themselves. If the abuse took place under the responsibility of a care organisation, then feelings of anger and mistrust exist towards the organisation, which in the eyes of the parents has failed in protecting their child. At the same time, the care organisation and the law authorities expect the parents to be able to put these feelings on hold for a while in order to work together as partners in supporting the client in the best way possible. There is a risk of the most important parties in the life of the client becoming disconnected, creating an extra hurdle in how those involved cope with the situation. This means that professional support is necessary for the parents and family in this complex situation!

In this chapter, the core aspects important for the professional to keep in mind during the conversations with parents are described. Four sessions are outlined in detail, and concrete guidelines are given for these conversations.

A help book for parents is also included in the SOS programme. In this help book, parents can keep a note of their experiences, feelings and questions, as well as reading background information. The contents of this help book should be adapted to the situation, and to the possibilities and limitation of the parents concerned. In Chapter 10, exercises for parents and caregivers are described, which the professional can use in putting together a suitable help book.

## 8.1 Core aspects for the support of parents

First, it is important for the professional to consider the complex dynamics of the situation for a family of a child with an intellectual disability who has been abused. The vulnerability of the child leads to protective reactions from the parents. This attitude of concern can be experienced as problematic and parents can, unfairly, receive the label 'difficult parents'. Parents of children with an intellectual disability often find it hard to let go of their child when they become an adult and to see them as an individual person, with their own feelings and emotions. The separation process is more difficult and can even stagnate, resulting in the parents and child staying together as one entity. Due to this, parents can see the abuse of their child as if they actually experienced it themselves – and their reactions can be just as strong.[2]

The build-up of powerlessness can also play a role: powerlessness in having a child with an intellectual disability, powerlessness regarding bringing the child up and possibly not being able to bring the child up themselves, powerlessness about a child being placed out of the home. On top of all this is the powerlessness felt about the abuse of the child.[3] Many parents experience a feeling of having to fight for the well-being of their child during their whole life.

In the case of an out-of-home placement, parents will have had to give their child, with feelings of sadness and powerlessness, into the hands of the care organisation. In the case of sexual abuse, parents can blame themselves for not having seen how unsafe their child was. In addition, if the abuse took place under the responsibility of the care organisation, they will feel anger and mistrust towards the care organisation which they entrusted with their child. It is important for the professional to be open and transparent in communicating with the parents, especially when mistakes have been made within the organisation. Recognising mistakes which have been made helps parents in coping with the situation after the abuse of their child.

Their own mortality can also be an issue for parents of adults with an intellectual disability. Parents worry about the safety of their child when they are no longer around and can become anxious about this. The professional should take this into consideration.

### 8.1.1 Family system and family culture

Before the conversations with the parents, the professional must do some research into the family system and the customs and values within the (family) culture. In order to identify the family system, the professional can form an image of the sociogram of the client who has been abused. This is important to ascertain which people in the system need support and who should be informed. In general, parents will always need support. The conversations are held with them, as described in this chapter. If the parents are divorced, or in the case of a blended family, it is very important to provide support for both mother and father. The professional should also find out whether or not parents have previously been confronted with abuse of a child.

For the other significant people in the sociogram of the victim, an estimate is made of their need for support/information. Sometimes a client will have elderly parents and the brother or sister will act as the contact person. In that case, it is important to offer this brother or sister support, alongside the parents. In some family cultures, it is not the parents but another family member who actually makes important decisions and has the most influence in family matters. In this case, this person should also be involved in the support programme. If the parents themselves have an intellectual disability, then it is important to adapt the information and conversations to their level. You can also consider involving the professional caregivers of the parents in the support programme.

Maybe the client is part, or used to be part, of a foster family and the foster parents are closely involved in the life of the client. It is then important to consider whether or not support should be provided for both the biological parents and the foster parents, and the way in which the sharing of tasks and the alignment between the foster organisation and the care organisation will be arranged. It is important to pay attention to the differences in resilience and perception during the support sessions, as a result of the various relationships and past histories of those involved.

Finally, it is important to know whether parents have their own (psychological) problems that the professional must consider during the conversations. It is also good to know whether or not the parent has experienced a traumatic situation in the past. If this is the case, then there is a chance that the abuse of the child will cause their personal story to come to the surface, along with the related trauma reactions.

### 8.1.2 Types of sexual abuse

It is possible that the client has suffered different types of sexual abuse, caused by different types of perpetrators. The client could have been abused by parents/carers, a family member, a family friend, staff at the care organisation, another client or a stranger. It is important that the professional realises that each of these different types of abuse can have an effect on how the conversation goes. If the sexual abuse was initiated within the family circle, then the consequences can reach far beyond the client and the parents themselves. This will also influence the stability of a family, as relationships with family and friends can come under pressure. When abuse was carried out by one of the parents then the conversations are only held with the parent who has not committed the abuse and with family members who have not committed the abuse. The (suspected) perpetrator is not involved in the SOS support programme!

The perpetrator is often well known to the victim. Research shows that sexual abuse is almost always committed by an acquaintance of the victim.[4] Due to the dependence of people with an intellectual disability, there is a large chance that this is someone known to the parents. This can cause confusion for parents in that they themselves can be so wrong about people they know and trusted. Parents can become unsure of themselves and suspicious, which not only influences the home situation, but also the circle of friends and the work environment. The professional must be alert to these reactions from parents. If they are not recognised, the suspicion can be taken as a motion of mistrust against the organisation where the client lives, for example. There is then a danger of misunderstanding and conflicts arising between parents and the care organisation.[5]

### 8.1.3 Creating safety

The professional talks to the parents about how the safety of their child can be guaranteed. In the first place, the victim should not be confronted with the (suspected) perpetrator. If this is an acquaintance or family member, taking safety precautions will be difficult to ensure. The practitioner should explicitly emphasise that this is essential for enabling the client to start coping with the situation.

The stress response system of the child will only be able to calm down when contact with the (suspected) perpetrator is avoided.

---

Attention must also be paid to taking safety precautions in school and work situations, during transport and free-time activities and in the use of social media!

---

The professional also emphasises that it is important for the child to restart the normal daily routines, such as reading a story or going to football training on Wednesday. Structure, regularity and predictability enhance the child's sense of safety and provide them with a feeling of being in control again, which helps to lessen the fear.[6]

This is, however, easier said than done in a situation in which the parents are confused and emotional. The parents can find it hard to set the boundaries because they feel sorry for their child and feel that their child has suffered already so much because of the trauma. They tend to be more indulgent and are unaware that the child needs these boundaries to feel safe again. However understandable this attitude is, it works counterproductively. In this time of upheaval, the child is dependent on the sense of security which the parents can offer!

Finally, the professional should discuss with the parents the way in which, alongside physical safety, an actual feeling of safety can be ensured. Structure in the daily routines is important, alongside providing safety messages. A safety message is a phrase or a statement in which the safety of the situation is emphasised, such as: 'It is safe here', 'I will make sure that everything will be OK here', 'Nothing can happen here'.

## 8.1.4 Reactions from parents

During the sessions with parents, the main focus is on the reactions of the parents to the abuse of their child. Parents are invited to talk about their own reactions during the conversations. Psychoeducation is provided by emphasising that after abuse has happened, a mass of emotions follow, including anger, sadness and disbelief.

One reaction which is often heard is that parents feel guilty about their child having been sexually abused. They think, 'I should have been there for my child' or 'I should have prevented it happening'. They think that they should have been able to recognise that abuse was taking place and realise what was happening to their child. These feelings of guilt can result in a belief that they are not a good mother or father. Parents, especially fathers, can hide or express their sadness, and possible feelings of guilt, with anger. This reaction often occurs and should not be underestimated.

As well as feeling guilty, denial can also play a role in the reactions of parents. They can doubt their child's story out of a sense of immunity; it is then important to inform parents that children rarely lie about sexual abuse. Parents can also deny that the abuse took place or trivialise the situation by saying that the damage is minimal. 'I was abused in the past and it didn't trouble me, so why should it trouble my child?' The professional can then react by saying that this is different for everybody and can ask how the parent managed to lessen the burden. This often provides an opening for a future conversation.

If the child has been abused by a family member or partner, feelings of betrayal and jealousy can also play a role. The parent can resent them having 'seduced' the other person behind their back. In a relationship of dependency, it is easier for the parent to be angry with the child than with the perpetrator. The parent (mostly subconsciously) assumes that the love from a child is unconditional, whereas it is much more difficult to win the love of a partner. Furthermore, uncertainty about separation can play a role when abuse has taken place within a family: 'My child will be moving out to live on their own soon, and if I don't choose the perpetrator's side, I will be left on my own'.

### *Tension from the past and the present*

During the conversations with parents, the professional must pay attention to the fact that the sexual abuse of the child acts as a trauma reminder for a parent who has been sexually abused themselves. The abuse of the child reminds the parent of their personal traumatic experience, which can cause overwhelming stress reactions from the parents.

It is important that the practitioner actively asks about this matter and validates and supports the parents and, if necessary, helps them to work on their own stabilisation.

Parents can also be troubled by seeing images of the abuse in their minds or re-experiencing it, especially during intimate moments with their partner. It is not uncommon for this to cause detachment and reproach between partners. This heightens the burden on the relationship between the parents, which is often already under pressure as a consequence of the serious incident which their child has experienced. It is important that the professional takes the initiative to talk about this and tells the parents that this is a reaction which often occurs, which will also disappear by itself. Talking about it will decrease the tension and meaning will be given to confusing and frightening reactions. In this way, space is created for bridging the feeling of distance which has arisen.

### 8.1.5 Reactions of the child

Providing psychoeducation on coping with trauma and stress reactions in children (and their parents) can help parents to understand their child's behaviour. It can also help them to explain common reactions in stress situations to their child and to be able to support the child more adequately. Useful practical knowledge about coping with stress reactions means that parents and children will (once again) experience more of a feeling of being in control of the situation. This will help to diminish feelings of fear and to enhance self-confidence. More information is given in Chapter 4 about stress reactions and coping with trauma.

#### *Questions*

Many parents ask themselves why their child hasn't (previously) told them about the abuse. It is important that the professional can discuss this question with the parents and highlight the various reasons the child may have had for not telling their parents about it. Children do not often tell others about abuse, because they are scared of how their parents will react. Sometimes children believe that the sexual abuse is their own fault and worry that they will not be believed, that they will be blamed and punished, or will have to leave home. Young children and children with a lower level of functioning are aware that the behaviour is wrong but are often unaware of whose fault it is. They are scared that they themselves are guilty for what has happened and are scared of getting into trouble. Perpetrators of sexual abuse often misuse this uncertainty.[7]

It is also possible that the child or their family has been threatened by the perpetrator to not talk to anyone about it. Shame can also mean that victims do not dare to tell anyone. If the perpetrator is someone within the circle of family or an acquaintance of the parents, then the child can be scared that this person will get into trouble. Children also say that they didn't tell anybody because they didn't want to sadden or hurt their parents.[8]

### *Boys*

If the child is a boy, who has been abused by a boy or a man, then the abuse can raise questions and concerns about the sexual identity of the boy, for both the parents and the client himself. Explanations in the form of psychoeducation are important in this case. Boys must be told that other boys are also sometimes abused by boys/men and that they are not alone in being victims of abuse. It is also important to say that the physical excitement which is felt at moments of abuse is not a sign of pleasure, but rather an autonomous reaction to sensations in the body. It is important that parents and their sons know that abuse has more to do with power and exercising control than with sex. Parents can tell their son that what has happened to him does not automatically mean that he is a homosexual and that this is no reason to be scared of homosexual men.[9]

Boys can also be abused by a woman. This often causes feelings of shame for boys, shame at not having been able to defend themselves against a woman. Moreover, feelings of uncertainty might have played a role: 'I am meant to enjoy this. So why does it trouble me so much?'

Psychoeducation on relationships of dependency and emotional and physical pressure is important in order to make the victim realise that they themselves are innocent.

### *Girls*

In the case of sexual abuse of girls, it is possible that the people around the child tell her that she herself was responsible for the abuse, because she was dressed in a sexy way or acted in a provocative, challenging manner. This can cause feelings of guilt and impurity within girls. The fact that a girl has lost her virginity, if emphasised by those around her, can strengthen feelings of guilt, impurity and damage.

Girls who have been abused by other girls or older women can start questioning their sexual identity. Just as is the case with boys, it is important to emphasise that this doesn't necessarily mean that they are now lesbian.

### *The consequences (of sexual abuse)*

Parents want to know how serious the consequences of the abuse of their child can be. The professional can discuss with the parents which factors influence the severity of the consequences. First, the relationship between the victim and the perpetrator is of importance. The stronger the attachment, the greater the risk of a trauma and there is a heightened chance that the child's ability to trust is damaged. The age of the child and how long the abuse has been taking place are also important factors. The younger the child was and the longer the duration of the abuse, the more damaging it will have been for the child.

Another important factor is the amount of violence which was used during the sexual abuse. The more violence used, the larger the child's trauma will be. A sexual activity which did not involve physical contact appears to be less traumatic for children. The context in which the abuse took place is also important. If the child has been made a victim at home, the consequences will be different from if the child became a victim outside of the trusted context.[10]

The reactions of others and the presence of an adult who can reassure them are eventually also an influence on the seriousness of the trauma (especially in the case of victims with an intellectual disability). If a child is not believed, or if they are accused or ignored, this will increase the trauma. Lack of a supportive adult will increase the feeling of loneliness, helplessness and worthlessness and will have a negative influence on the severity of the trauma.[11]

Parents often ask the question: 'Will my own child become a perpetrator?' or 'Will my child also abuse other children themselves?' The professional can explain that this certainly does not have to be the case and that normalising and supporting their child's sexual development will play an important role in this issue.

---

Conversations with parents take place to discuss which factors play a role in the situation of their own child and what these mean for the child.

---

### 8.1.6 Dealing with the child's stress reactions

An important part of the conversations with parents is the way in which parents react towards their child. Parents have many questions about this. The most important thing for parents to do when the child has been abused is to be there for their child, to support them and to assume that the child is telling the truth.[12] Well-meant advice such as, 'Try not to think about it' or 'Try to forget about it' often affects the child's ability to cope. Negative and trivialising reactions to the abuse should also be avoided. Reactions such as, 'Why didn't you try to stop him?' or 'You must not have understood it properly', do not help the child to move on and can confirm their own feelings of guilt.[13]

Parents help the child in the best way by ensuring that the child can express their feelings to them or to another adult. What also helps is being able to retreat for a while and to be comforted without words. Parents should realise that they mean a lot to their child by simply being there for them and supporting them. They are not required to take the pain away; this just isn't possible. Dealing with the situation together and giving the abuse a place between all the good and bad things in life is what it is all about.

If the police interview still has to take place and the child has to give a statement, the professional will instruct the parents about the way in which the child will be spoken to. The practitioner may advise the parents not to talk about the facts (who, what, where, when and how) and not to ask too many questions concerning the facts. Parents can listen to their child's story, support their child emotionally and emphasise that the child is now safe (if this is actually the case). Parents can also tell their child that it is a very good thing that they have told their story.

The professional should talk to the parents about how they can adapt their reactions to the situation. It is important to support parents in learning to regulate their own emotions in the presence of the child, and in this way to provide a feeling of safety and to act as role models for their child. If victims see their parents being overwhelmed when they talk about the abuse, then the children will not want to talk about it anymore. Based on a feeling of responsibility for the well-being of their parents they will then play down their own feelings and pain.[14]

If parents do become emotional during a conversation with the child, it is important that they explain that the child is not at fault and is not the cause of mum and dad crying. They can explain that they are angry about the situation or at the person who did this to the child.

---

It is essential to talk to parents about the best ways in which to regulate their own emotions at times that they feel overwhelmed; for example, walking away from the situation, going for a stroll or focusing on their breathing.

---

Parents have to let their child know that they are never the guilty party when it comes to having been sexually abused. Sometimes a child is sexually abused while doing something that the parents had forbidden them to do. Going to visit the new neighbour, for example, when the parents had said they weren't allowed to do so. Parents can then be clear about the fact that the child didn't listen properly, but they must also be clear that the child did not cause the sexual abuse.[15]

It is important to emphasise to parents that it is not sensible to threaten revenge on the perpetrator in the presence of the child. This could increase the child's fear that the perpetrator will harm the child or the parents and that the child, on top of what has already happened, awaits even more threats. They may be scared of losing their parents, if they become injured or imprisoned.

It is typical in cases of sexual abuse that the child does not have control over the situation. It is important to reinstate a feeling of being in control. Parents can do this by letting their child make their own decisions in keeping with the situation and with their possibilities. Providing the opportunity of making (small or larger) choices can give the child the feeling that they can influence the situation again.

### *Time-in*

During the sessions with parents, specific attention should be paid to the fact that children who have experienced abuse often have the tendency to test the boundaries (again). The professional explains to parents how to react to this in a suitable way, and that this reaction is caused by a feeling of being unsafe, instead of by a behavioural problem or disobedience. The professional explains that, at such times, it is not a good idea to give the child a 'time-out' (by sending them to their room, for example), which parents may be used to doing. Putting a traumatised child in a place on their own increases the feeling of unsafety and isolation.[16] The practitioner gives parents the advice that in this case it is better to give them a 'time-in': let the child sit next to them to calm down. This lessens the feelings of unsafety and helps much more than a time-out in these situations.

### 8.1.7 Other members of the family

It is important to think about the influence which the abuse has on other family members. Have other family members been informed? In which way are the conversations with brothers and sisters conducted? What role can the parents play in talking to them? It is important to state the importance of talking about the abuse situation in an open and honest way within the family. In the sessions with parents, the professional can discuss the best ways in which to talk to the other children in the family about what has happened and how they can adapt what they say to suit the level of development and the present situation of the child.

### 8.1.8 The surrounding environment

Another important theme in the sessions with parents is the reactions from those around them. In general, people find it hard to react to an incident of sexual abuse. Friends of parents often do not dare to ask about it. Some people say the wrong things or make rude jokes.

Common reactions are:

- The people in the surrounding environment do not recognise the psychological impact of what has happened.
- The people in the surrounding environment give the parents a feeling of guilt ('Did you, as a mother, really not notice anything?').

- The people in the surrounding environment trivialise what has happened ('At least your child is still alive').
- The people in the surrounding environment do not seek contact with parents ('We thought it best to leave you in peace. You've already got so much going on in your life').
- The people in the surrounding environment tell the parents what they would do if they were in their shoes, and how they would react. This often results in advice which does not help the parents.

These reactions can cause parents to feel very lonely. The professional talks to parents about the reactions from people around them – what has helped them and how they deal with annoying reactions.

Feelings of shame also play a role for parents in telling others about what has happened.[17] What do parents tell and to whom? It can help to look for concrete ways in which they can talk about the subject with other important people in their lives.

---

It is important to emphasise to parents the strong points you see in the child and in the family, and to highlight the strength of the support which has been initiated by the SOS programme.

---

## 8.1.9 The coping process of the parents

During the conversations with the parents, the professional must make sure that they do not only talk about the child. There is a chance that the parents and the practitioner will be tempted to do so, due to avoidance reactions.

The parents' own way of coping with the situation must emphatically be discussed during the conversations!

The parents should be supported in finding a balance between looking after their child and looking after themselves. It is important to talk to parents about how looking after themselves is essential in order to be able to look after their child properly. It is also important that the professional checks whether there are enough people around them to whom they can express their feelings and whether or not they actually make use of this possibility. If necessary, the practitioner thinks, together with the parents, about where adequate sources of support can be found and how they can be approached.

## 8.2 The SOS programme for parents

The starting point for the SOS programme is that the parents are aware of the fact that their child has been abused. If this is not the case, then a separate bad news conversation will be held before the first session.

The SOS programme for parents consists of the joint session and three separate sessions for parent. The contents of these sessions are described here.

### 8.2.1 Attitude aspects

During the sessions, the professional takes an open, equal and supportive approach. It is important to act as a clear role model for the way in which issues are described, and to show capability and active involvement. The practitioner can use a (appropriate) sense of humour to make sure that the atmosphere of the sessions does not become too fraught.

The professional keeps the parents updated, including in between the sessions. Send an email or call if new facts become known which are also important for the parents. This allows you to break the feeling of isolation. In everything, it is important that the practitioner honours the agreements which have been made! People who have experienced serious incidents have an increased need for predictability and reliability. This is necessary to be able to feel in control of the situation again.

### 8.2.2 Preparation by the professional

Before the sessions, the professional should research the family system/situation and the customs and values which apply within this (family) culture. As mentioned previously, it is important to be aware of the sociogram of the client: who are the significant others in their life?

### 8.2.3 Time and place of the sessions with the parents

The first conversation with parents should ideally take place on the same day as the abuse is disclosed, or otherwise as soon as possible afterwards. The first conversation is led by the professional who is responsible and preferably takes place at the home of the parents. This is a well-known and safe environment which makes it easier for parents to talk openly. In this way, the professional will be able to form a reliable view of the parents, the client and their symptoms and needs.

The next talk with the parents is one week after the first conversation, three weeks after the second conversation and a follow-up conversation eight weeks after the first conversation. The third session is a joint session for the parents, the client, (representatives from) the care team, the manager and the professional. The guideline is that each session lasts about one-and-a-half hours.

### 8.2.4 Structure of the sessions

The professional arranges four sessions with parents/carers. The first contact takes place as soon as possible, preferably within a week of the disclosure/discovery (and after the minimum fact interview). The second session takes place about one week later. The third session is a joint session, in which the client, their system and the professional caregivers involved share their experiences and (learn) to communicate with each other about what has happened. This joint session is held about one month after the start of the programme. After eight weeks there is a follow-up meeting for the parents.

When conducting the SOS programme, the professional must realise that there is no fixed content for the conversations. This depends on the individual situation of parents and which subjects arise at which moments.

The subjects can be clustered into three main themes which are covered in every session:

- talking about the sexual abuse
- emotional support for parents
- providing psychoeducation.

Talking about sexual abuse gives the professional and the parents the opportunity to reconstruct and order the incident of abuse. Emotional support for parents is given by providing a listening ear and being there for the parents in this time of upheaval. Naming, discussing and giving meaning to thoughts and feelings which parents have regarding the abuse is essential here. In addition, providing psychoeducation is a central part of the SOS programme. By obtaining information about trauma and coping with trauma and stress reactions and how to deal with them, parents will find understanding, control and a feeling of certainty about being able to cope with the situation.

### 8.2.5 Using the help book for parents

The help book is put together by the professional before the first session and can be added to after each session. The pages of the help book are printed and put together in a folder. A tab page 'letters and forms' is added, so that parents can add correspondence and other forms/information to the folder. The practitioner gives the parents instructions about how to use the help book:

*'This help book is for you. You can use it to collect and store information about the abuse. There are various tab-pages in the folder. Behind the first tab-page, you will see a number of forms, on which you can write down your own thoughts and feelings about the abuse. You can also keep a note here of feelings and questions which arise in between the sessions and which are important to talk about together.*

*'There is also a page on which you can both keep a note of your own symptoms. This may seem exaggerated, but it does prove to be useful. The strange thing about symptoms is that, when you have had them for a long period of time, you can get used to them and don't really notice them anymore. And we want to know how your symptoms are and if they are changing. That's why it's good to keep a note of them. It is, of course, not compulsory to fill in the form, but I do recommend it.*

*'Behind the second tab-page you can keep letters and forms, for example letters about the police statement, information from the police, and so on.*

*'Behind the last tab-page, you will find information about various issues which we have talked about during the sessions, for example about common reactions displayed by children who have been abused. Maybe you would like to add to it with information from the internet or which you have received from other people.'*

## 8.3 Sessions for parents

The SOS programme for parents consists of four parent sessions, one of which is a joint session. As mentioned previously, there is no fixed table of contents. The subjects are adapted to suit the parent's individual situation. The professional makes sure that the three main themes are covered in each session. These themes are: talking about the sexual abuse, emotional support for parents and providing psychoeducation.

### 8.3.1 Parent session 1: as soon as possible

What is needed?

- SOS handbook
- The help book for parents
- Appropriate worksheets, for example:
    - 'Talking about sexual abuse' (Chapter 10)
    - 'Thoughts and feelings' (Chapter 10)
    - 'Sexual abuse' (Chapter 10).

Duration of the session: 90 minutes.

#### *Talking about sexual abuse*

During the first session, listening to the parents' story and talking about the sexual abuse is the main theme. Parents are often overwhelmed by the whole situation. This is expressed by asking practical questions about what has happened. Feelings and emotions often arise at a later stage. It is important to take the time to listen properly to the parents' story.

The following questions can help to get the conversation started:

- How did you hear about the abuse?
- How did you find hearing about it in that way?
- What have you heard exactly?
- Which feelings does this cause?
- How did you react?
- Do you have any questions about what has happened?
- Did it surprise you?
- Did you notice anything in your child's behaviour?
- If you look back, do things fall into place?

If possible, add to the information which parents have.

### *Emotional support for the parents*

- Have you already spoken to your child or seen them?
- How did that go?
- Did your child say anything about it?
- Did you say anything about it?
- Are you pleased with how this went?
- Looking back, what would you have rather done?
- What was difficult?
- What was easier than you thought?
- Which concerns do you have about your child?
- And how are you feeling?
- How are you sleeping, eating and relaxing?
- What do you notice about yourself? And about each other?

Usually, it helps to explain that men and women often react differently to these sorts of situations and due to this can clash with each other. You can use the cliché of how women endlessly want to talk about things and are emotional, and how men just want to get on and do things and not talk about it too much. Experience teaches that this works in a forgiving way and lightens the tone of the conversation.

You can also ask whether or not they can talk to each other about it and which feelings this creates. Don't forget to ask both parents. Their reactions can be extremely different.

### *Psychoeducation on talking about sexual abuse and stress reactions*

After providing space for the parents' own experience and story, it is a good idea to provide information about the reactions which parents can expect, in both themselves and their child. Talk about stress symptoms and explain that not only the child is troubled by these, but also others in the surrounding environment. Ask what they recognise in themselves, in others and in their child.

Explain that after-effects are normal in situations such as these. These are normal reactions to abnormal events. It is a sort of adapting reaction from our system which is trying to cope with the situation, and this will stop by itself. It is actually a healthy reaction and it would have been of more concern if the parents weren't troubled by the situation at all.

Explain that parents often see the incident of abuse in their minds and ask if they are experiencing this as well.

You can also talk about questions which the parents ask, such as: What do I tell my child? What will I tell the school? What will I tell the family?

It is possible that agreements should be made about issues such as preparing the statement or police interview.

### *End of the session*

At the end of the conversation, an assessment takes place with the parents as to whether or not safety agreements need to be made, for example regarding contact with the (suspected) perpetrator. Discuss practical issues which the parents may want to talk about, such as how to deal with the use of the telephone, internet and social media, and discuss agreements which need to be made with the school, day care centre and whether taxi transport should be considered. Introduce the help book and give this to the parents.

At the end of the conversation, ask how the parents look back on the session and if there was anything which moved them or helped them.

Let the parents fill in the 'Session evaluation' form (see Chapter 10) for the first session. Ask if they missed certain elements in the session or if you can do anything else for them.

Tell them that you are impressed by the efforts which theyare making for their child and that you are keen to work with them further.

At the end of the first session, an arrangement is made for the second session to be held one week later.

Give parents the worksheet 'Session preparation' (see Chapter 10).

### 8.3.2 Parent session 2: after a week

What is needed?

- SOS handbook
- Help book for the parents
- Appropriate worksheets, for example:
    - 'Dos and don'ts for talking about sexual abuse with a victim' (Chapter 10)
    - 'My fault or not?' (Chapter 10)
    - 'Looking after yourself test' (Chapter 10).

Duration of the session: 90 minutes.

#### *Talking about sexual abuse*

One week after the first parent session, the professional will visit the parents again. In the second session the present situation is discussed. The parents are asked about any changes in the last week. New information is organised and the experience and emotions of the parents are talked about. How is this experience now? Which emotions are in the foreground?

### *Emotional support for the parents*

In this second conversation, attention can be paid to the daily routine of the parents. Are they succeeding in regaining this? How is work going? Where are they experiencing hurdles? Are the parents able to look after themselves properly?

Parents often say, 'I'm not important, my child is important now'. If they react in this way, it is good to emphasise the fact that parents cannot look after their child properly if they don't look after themselves. The following comparison can help here:

*'Have you ever flown? At the beginning of the flight the safety instructions are given in case anything happens. An explanation is given that in an emergency it is important for parents to put on their safety mask first, before helping their child. If the parents fall unconscious due to lack of oxygen, they can do nothing to help their child. You are now in a similar situation. If you don't look after yourself first (and put your own oxygen mask on), then you cannot look after your child properly.'*

It is also a good idea to talk about the parents' relationship. Can they support one another? How is the intimacy and sexuality in the relationship? Has this been influenced by what the child has experienced?

### *Psychoeducation on talking about stress symptoms and support needs*

In this second conversation, the reactions of the child can be discussed. Fill in the worksheet 'Child/client post-traumatic stress symptoms checklist' together (Chapter 10).

### *Preparation of the third session*

During this session, the third, joint session is discussed and preparations are made with the parents. The preparation during the second session consists of brainstorming with the parents about what could help their child:

- What positive things can the parents say to the child?
- Which characteristics do the parents value in their child and can these help the child? Forexample: 'Do you remember

when you got your swimming certificate? Then you were brave and you can be brave again now!'

- What would the parents like to do with the child in the future?
- What do the parents wish the child for the future?

It is important to emphasise the importance of parents expressing hope and perspective in the joint session. The aim of the third, joint session can be explained as follows:

*'In the joint session we will talk with all those involved about what has happened. You will be present, together with your child and the child's professional caregiver (and the manager, if the abuse took place under the responsibility of a care organisation). It is important to pay attention to what has happened together, because everyone is shocked, and to learn to talk about what has happened.*

*'During this session, your child will be encouraged to talk about the ways in which the people around them can help. It is important to tell your child, with all of those present, that it is not their fault and that you are supporting them. Together with the child, we will make sure that the child starts to feel better again. You can name the positive characteristics of the child, which they can use in the following period. Then a joint "Together we are strong" exercise is done with all those present.'*

### *End of the session*

The second session ends by talking about what is now important for the parents. At the end of the conversation, the help book is looked through together and added to with the information which has been discussed in the second session.

At the end of the conversation, ask how the parents experienced the session and if there is anything that moved them or helped them. Ask if they missed certain elements in the session or if you can do anything else for them. Let the parents fill this in in the 'Session evaluation' form (see Chapter 10).

Finally, an arrangement is made for the third joint session to be held three weeks after the second session.

### 8.3.3 Parent session 3: joint session – after three weeks

A joint session is held three weeks after the second session, in which the child, the parents/family, the caregivers and the professional are present. This conversation is held in a place which is safe for the child, in the presence of significant others in the life of the child. You start by having a snack together, for example a cup of tea and a biscuit. This is important because the food and drink can lessen the fear and help to restore and improve the relationships.

What is needed?

- The SOS handbook
- The presence of manager/team leader as co-leader of the meeting
- Something to eat and drink
- Flip-chart or whiteboard
- Worksheet 'Together we are strong' (see client's help book)
- Equipment with which to do the 'Together we are strong' exercise, such as drawing/craft supplies.

Depending on the client's taste you can also use glitter, stars, photos, a computer and so on.

After the session you give the help book back. Agree with the caregivers how and when they will help the client.

Duration of the session: approximately two hours in total. The joint discussion takes about one hour. Then there is an informal meeting with everyone involved; the aim of this is a feeling of togetherness, restarting communication, getting back to normal life again.

#### *The start of the session*

Tell those involved about the session:

*'Today we are going to talk to each other about what has happened. This is important because everyone is shocked by what happened. By talking to each other about it, we can help each other.'*

Explain the structure of the session in concrete terms:

*'We are here together in...'s room. We will begin by drinking a cup of tea or coffee with a biscuit. Then I (or the name of someone else) will lead the discussion and make sure that it goes well. When we have finished talking, we will make something together. After that we will talk some more and then we'll end the session together.'*

### *Talking about the sexual abuse*

The professional, or the manager who is present, begins by giving a short description of what has happened. If the police interview has already been held, it will be possible to say more than if it has yet to take place. A timeline and/or sociogram may be used to tell the story.

### *Psychoeducation on stress reactions and support needs*

Subsequently the psychoeducation part of the session takes place, during which the professional explains that everyone is very shocked by the situation and reacts in their own way:

*'Everyone is very shocked by what has happened and each person reacts in their own way. You may be angry, scared or sad. Let's hear how everyone has reacted.'*

The person who leads the conversation then gives those present, one at a time, the chance to tell how they have reacted and this is written on the flip-chart. For clients who cannot read or write you can work with smileys to communicate the reactions of those involved.

It is important that the reactions of parents and professionals are prepared during previous meetings. The joint session is intended as a support session for the client. Parents and caregivers can describe their reactions in short and emphasise the fact that it is good that the client has told others about what was troubling them. The parents and caregivers can explain that it is never the child's fault that something like this happens. They can also explicitly say that it is not the child's fault that adults are feeling sad now. For example:

*'I was angry/scared/...'*

Then tell the client:

*'You did well to tell others about it (if this is how it has been discovered) and how you are dealing with it now. It is not your fault that I'm feeling like this. It is the perpetrator's fault. They were at fault, not you.'*

It is important to steer the content of the discussion in this direction and, if necessary, to add this information yourself. Clients must be relieved of guilt and must be empowered! If other participants in the discussion require extra support, this should take place at a different moment.

### *Together we are strong!*

The client is asked how they are feeling now and if there is anything else they would like to say. The person who led the discussion with the client in session 2 helps the client (if necessary using the help book) to express what is on their mind. Attention is paid to practical issues, safety and reactions to what parents and professionals have said. In addition, attention is paid to the wishes of the client regarding the type of support during the next few weeks. What is the best way to help the client and with which activities? What does the client like doing and what helps best?

The most appropriate 'Together we are strong' activity is chosen, for example:

- 'Together we are strong – the plaster' (Section 6.3)
- 'Together we are strong – the message' (Section 6.3)
- 'Together we are strong – the song' (Section 6.3)
- 'Together we are strong – music' (Section 7.4).

The 'Together we are strong' activity is meant to break through the isolation which people can feel after experiencing something traumatic. Above all, it is meant to let clients experience that everyone is working together and help to make dealing with the abuse bearable. The professional introduces the exercise and explains, in a way adapted to the level of the client, that abuse hurts.

### *The end of the session – talking about what we thought of the discussion*

At the end of the session, those involved are asked what they thought of the session. You can choose to do this with everyone involved or only with the client. The choice depends on how the discussion goes, the characteristics of the client and of the parents (are there problems relating to the parents, are there intense emotions and so on?). Can the client talk about this with the other people present or will the client benefit more from talking about it individually with you? Write in the client's help book (or let the client write) about the conversation and what they thought of it. Put the joint activity, or a photo of it, in the client's help book and let them take it home with them.

### *What next?*

Agree and write down who will support the client in the following weeks and at which times. Tell the client that these people are going to support them and that the client doesn't have to visit the professional during the next few weeks. Say that an appointment will be made after a while to see how the client is feeling and how they are being supported. Make an actual appointment and write this down in the help book.

Then make a link back to the daily life of the client, for example by talking about the rest of the day.

## 8.3.4 Parent session 4: follow-up – after two months

What is needed?

- SOS handbook
- Help book for the parents
- Appropriate worksheets, for example:
    - 'Secondary traumatic stress checklist' (Chapter 10)
    - 'Support from people around you' (Chapter 10)
    - 'SOS evaluation form' (Chapter 10).

Duration of the session: 90 minutes.

### *Talking about sexual abuse*

After two months, the professional visits the parents again. The situation at the present moment is discussed during this follow-up:

- How are the parents and the child doing?

Attention is paid to the experience and emotions of the parents:

- What is their experience at the moment?
- Which emotions are in the foreground?
- Which questions do the parents have?

### *Psychoeducation on secondary traumatising*

Possible PTSD symptoms of the child can be discussed with the parents (if this has been done in session 2) using the 'Child/client post-traumatic stress symptoms checklist' (Chapter 10). Whether or not therapy is necessary for the child can be discussed. For example, EMDR (eye movement desensitisation and reprocessing), a non-verbal type of therapy which is aimed at lessening the symptoms quickly. Other forms of therapy can also be discussed, such as behaviour therapy, play therapy, creative therapy or psychomotor therapy. Which sort of therapy is most appropriate will depend on the type of symptoms and the child's character.

### *Emotional support for the parents*

During the follow-up, it is important to pay attention to symptoms which the parent may be suffering and to referral for possible further professional help.

### *End of the session and evaluation*

The SOS programme is evaluated with the parents using the 'SOS evaluation form' (Chapter 10). What did the parents think about the help provided? What do they still need in order to be able to cope with the situation?

## SUMMARY

Incidents of sexual abuse do not only have consequences for the child themselves, but also for the people around them. The support for parents is discussed in this chapter as being an essential part of the SOS programme. The emphasis is on how parents cope after abuse and on informing them about the child's coping process. The parents coping with the situation in a good way is essential for the child to be able to cope with the situation.

Various core aspects, which are of importance for the professional in the conversations with parents, are explained in this chapter. Descriptions of system aspects regarding families of children with an intellectual disability are given, alongside various aspects which parents can be confronted with concerning sexual abuse.

Four sessions are described, during which the three important themes are discussed, these being: talking about sexual abuse, emotional support for parents and providing psychoeducation for parents.

The main focus is on the fact that people with a disability are dependant, more so than others, on the reactions of those around them in coping with the abuse.

Chapter 9

# SUPPORT OF HEALTHCARE PROFESSIONALS WORKING WITH VICTIMS OF SEXUAL ABUSE

## Introduction

The way in which people with an intellectual disability cope with experiences of sexual abuse greatly depends on the reactions of significant others in their lives, such as parents and other family members, and is also influenced by the reactions of professional caregivers.[1] Working with victims of sexual abuse who have an intellectual disability, and with their social system, is a special area of expertise. Issues such as guilt, belief and disbelief can inhibit the adequate functioning of professional caregivers and the healthcare team concerned.

In this chapter, specific attention is paid to the processes of splitting, transference and countertransference, which are unavoidable in situations of abuse. practitioners should be aware of the enormous impact on the working environment and on the quality of support for the client and their system, if too little attention is paid to contradictory feelings and the uncertainty of colleagues about how to deal with the situation properly.

Four sessions are described in this chapter in which practitioners help the professional caregivers involved in supporting a client who has suffered sexual abuse. The sessions focus emphatically on the support – and not the treatment – of the victim (and their system) in their daily living environment. Alongside attention to practical guidelines for supporting the client, specific attention is also paid to the support of the healthcare professionals in their own process and that of their colleagues. Adequate daily support for a client is only possible if the healthcare professionals involved are able to order and discuss their own experiences and perceptions. The healthcare professional acts as a role model for the client here. Guidelines are also given for stabilising the situation, making an inventory of the sexual abuse, providing emotional support and the psychoeducation of the healthcare professionals involved. Practical exercises are provided which the practitioner can use to discuss various issues during the support of the professional caregivers involved.

## 9.1 Core aspects in the support of healthcare professionals involved

### 9.1.1 A safe and reliable environment for the client

The most basic requirement for the support of victims of sexual abuse is a safe environment. A basic requirement for a safe environment is that contact between the client and the (suspected) perpetrator is prevented.[2, 3, 4] A safe environment minimises risky situations. Agreements should be made about measures which can be taken to limit risks. It is the professional's task to make sure that these agreements are synchronised with all of the client's social environments, at home, school, work, free time and in the residential accommodation (and during transport between these places). It is essential that the client is aware of these safety measures.

However, safety does not only consist of physical safety; the perception of safety (also known as psychological safety) of the victim is also essential. This form of safety is not only achieved by the feeling of being in control of the outside world, but also by the feeling of being in control of one's own emotions. Issues which remind a person of the abuse can give rise to physical and emotional reactions, which undermine the feeling of safety. Sometimes a victim will understand what has happened, but reactions are more often totally subconscious (definitely in the case of people with an intellectual disability) making them even more frightening. In the perception of these victims, the threat of danger is everywhere and they feel that nowhere is safe.[5]

In order to create a feeling of safety, a direct attitude ('this is how we are going to do things') is required by the caregivers.

The caregiver needs to simply 'be there' and radiate peace. The caregiver should provide frequent safety messages, repeat again and again that the abuse is over now and that the victim is safe in the here and now. It is recommended to agree on a code or sign, which the client can use to express themselves if things aren't going well. The caregiver can then respond to this by providing a safety message or help by providing distractions or relaxation.

*Recognisable and predictable*

A safe and reliable environment also means that the surroundings are recognisable and predictable. The client needs steady beacons which offer a firm foundation. In this way the victim can get back to daily life again. Stress factors should be reduced as much as possible (see Chapter 4).

A reliable environment also means that healthcare professionals do what they say, and say what they do. Don't make any promises that you are not sure of being able to keep, and inform the client about what is happening as much as possible! It is the task of the practitioner to make sure that healthcare professionals and the client's system work together. This prevents confusion in the client. Open communication and good synchronisation are key here.

It is important that healthcare professionals who work with victims of sexual abuse are aware of their approach to closeness and touch. Some clients experience touch as being very threatening, others will continuously ask for touch. The practitioner should ensure a support style which is adapted to the needs of the individual client. Attention should be paid to the vulnerability of the client and socially acceptable boundaries and it may be necessary to offer alternative physical behaviour.

### 9.1.2 Talking with the client about the sexual abuse

It was often advised in the past to let the client take the initiative to talk about sexual abuse. Victims would talk about it themselves, when they were ready to do so. Experience and research[6] have taught us that this is not the case, and definitely not for children and people with an intellectual disability. Reconstructing and reorganising details of the incident, and expressing thoughts and feelings in a safe context, can be of enormous help for clients in regaining the feeling that they are in control of their lives. Talking about the incident means that it can be 'psychologically ruminated'. In time, the intensity of the feelings will lessen, the sharp edges will soften.[7] As a result, avoidance behaviour is reduced and false cognitions ('It was my fault', 'Men are not to be trusted' and so on) about the sexual abuse can be corrected. This gives opportunities for learning adequate coping skills.

Talking about sexual abuse is difficult and there are extra obstacles in talking about sexual abuse with victims with an intellectual disability. On the one hand, this is due to the fact that this group of people often have more difficuty expressing things in words – or even at all. It is also more difficult for them to see current feelings, thoughts and behaviour in relation to the sexual abuse. On the other hand, healthcare professionals (and parents) around the victim often also have their own intense reactions: How is it possible that someone abuses this vulnerable person? How could it have happened under our noses? Why didn't we see the signs?

The reaction to the sexual abuse from the surrounding environment is of great importance for the coping process of the victim. It is the task of the professional, together with the professional caregivers, to reconstruct and reorganise the incident and the perception of it. There must be sufficient opportunities created to release personal emotions and tensions out of the client's presence.

The professional caregivers should be aware of the importance of reacting in a calm and open manner to a client who is a victim of sexual abuse. An intense emotional reaction of a listener often leads to victims stopping to tell their story, leaving out or taking back the worst details in order to protect the caregiver. It is also possible that clients with an intellectual disability get the message that the emotions of the other person are the only proper emotions. As a result, the client may take on the emotions of the caregiver and not be able to discover and express their own emotions.

In addition, caregivers should be aware of the influence of their own expectations and the necessity of adapting these to the perception of the client.

Depending on the protocols which are applicable in the healthcare organisations concerned, it is important to pay attention to minimum fact interviews and the possibility of a police interview while talking about the sexual abuse (see Section 3.4.2).

### 9.1.3 Getting back to normal life

It is important that caregivers keep to the normal daily routines as much as possible. These routines enhance the feeling of safety, give a feeling of control and help to lessen anxiety. It is important that a victim sees that the regular daily structure of the time before the abuse simply continues as it was, such as eating and sleeping on time, reading a story, going to football training on Wednesdays.[8] If there is a loss of skills in the area of self-reliance, this should in the first case be respected and interpreted as being part of the general upset. Don't pressurise the client to do the same things independently as they did before the abuse. Caregivers should have an eye for the way in which the client function changes as a result of the trauma symptoms. They can take over certain care tasks for the client if necessary and let the client experience the feeling of being looked after. When the client has regained their sense of balance, the former skills and support level can be reinstated step by step in mutual agreement.

Caregivers should be aware of the way in which the client function changes as a result of trauma symptoms. A client may be able to do some things one day, and the next day be unable to perform the same actions. This should be supported in a flexible way.

#### *Positive feeling*

During the support for a victim of sexual abuse, it is important to maintain a healthy balance between specific support and continuity of the normal programme.[9, 10, 11] The coping process after abuse means that the abuse is given a place between the positive and the negative things in life. For this reason, it is important that the victim, alongside this intense incident and everything involved with it, also experiences pleasant and beautiful times. Such experiences can also provide distraction after the abuse. It is important that the client has positive experiences to reinstate the feeling of self-worth and a positive body image. Physical activities (having a bath, beauty treatments, make-up and so on) are of invaluable worth here.

Physical exercise is also important. Intense sport and exercise releases endorphins, which increase the victim's general feeling of well-being in a healthy way. Physical activity also creates physical tiredness, which enhances sleep. Many victims of sexual abuse are troubled by sleeping disorders. There should be specific attention for reinstating a healthy sleeping pattern. Encourage steady day and night rhythms and doing relaxing activities before going to bed.

#### *The right balance*

Too much focus on getting back to normal life can give victims the idea that they aren't being taken seriously. This can get in the way of the coping process. Too much specific attention for the abuse, however, can work in a stigmatising way and obstruct the ability to get back to normal life. Emphasising the feeling of being weak and helpless can lower resilience. A good balance between getting back to normal life on the one hand, and paying specific attention to the abuse on the other hand, requires a good synchronisation between the professional, the client's system, pedagogic staff and possible therapists.

### 9.1.4 Dealing with trauma reactions of the client

Good support for a client after a severe incident consists of understanding and acceptance of the reactions of the victim.[12] Sexual abuse generally entails the abuse of trust and disrespect of boundaries, meaning that the victim often no longer trusts people in his or her environment. Many victims (some for a long time) test whether people can be trusted by demonstrating behaviour which could damage the relationship. 'Difficult' behaviour displayed by people with a disability is often an expression of emotions which they otherwise find difficult to express.

The professional should provide psychoeducation for the team about stress reactions and coping behaviour. Diverse exercises are described in Chapter 10 for this purpose. Caregivers are helped in this way to see emotional and problematic behaviour in a trauma context. It is a normal stress reaction to an abnormal situation, or it is learnt coping behaviour which the client has used to help them survive the sexual abuse.

By teaching the caregivers to look at the behaviour through trauma spectacles, they will be more able to react to the behaviour in an understanding way and to accept it for what it is. Give the client control and direction over their own life, wherever possible. Let a client think for themselves and make their own decisions. Caregivers look after basic needs and in this way give the client the feeling that they are being looked after. If there are somatic issues, physical symptoms should be taken seriously and not trivialised.

This does not mean though that undesirable behaviour should always be tolerated. Negative behaviour must be stopped without rejecting the person themselves. Offer the client concrete alternatives for negative behaviour.

Caregivers should be conscious of the importance of using a 'time-in' instead of a 'time-out' for undesirable behaviour. Undesirable behaviour after intense life events is generally the result of a feeling of unsafety, meaning that the client actually requires extra care and closeness and a reliable care figure who helps to regulate their behaviour. A time-out in which the client is placed in a separate place works in a counterproductive way and leads to an increase in feelings of unsafety and problematic behaviour.

### 9.1.5 Dealing with stress reactions from parents

Although the practitioner plays an important role in the SOS programme in the support of parents/guardians of a client who has been sexually abused, this does not mean that the daily professional caregivers do not also play a role here. In contacts between healthcare professionals and parents, it is important that the healthcare professional takes the initiative. Daily caregivers should not only ask about the client, but also about the perceptions of the parents. The aim is to support the client together.

The professional caregiver should realise that parents also display stress reactions, and must see unreasonable or angry behaviour within this context and perceive it as such. An understanding attitude with regard to the impact of sexual abuse for parents of the client helps here. It is the task of the professional to provide psychoeducation for the caregivers about the implications of sexual abuse of people with an intellectual disability, trauma and coping with trauma. Diverse exercises are described in Chapter 10 for this purpose.

### 9.1.6 Splitting

There is rarely clear evidence to be found in situations of sexual abuse. This results in the way in which emotions, loyalties and interpretations play an important role in situations of (suspected) sexual abuse. It is understandable that the sexual abuse of a client by an unknown person will give rise to different processes from a situation in which a colleague is the (suspected) perpetrator. If a (suspected) perpetrator appears to be a colleague, then healthcare professionals will often feel even more confused. Which of my colleagues can I still trust? But also: How should we deal with distance and closeness with regard to the clients? Cuddling a client suddenly becomes an emotionally charged topic.[13]

A (suspicion of) sexual abuse in clients among themselves brings specific support needs for both the clients involved and for the healthcare professionals who work with them.

Splitting describes a disruptive division between 'believers' and 'non-believers'. This division can arise within a healthcare team, within the organisation (managers – team of managers – directors), between organisations involved (healthcare organisation – family guardian – institution), with the family of the (suspected) victim and/or perpetrator (parents – team of parents – managers), but also in the wider social context. Camps form, each concentrating on their own problems. This drives the parties further apart, consciously or subconsciously. This complex dynamic leads to those involved acting on the basis of their own emotions, which can lead to risky situations where disclosures and signs from victims are not taken seriously and/or are interpreted in the wrong way. Suspected victims are sometimes not believed, suspected perpetrators are sometimes stigmatised unjustifiably or actual perpetrators are not recognised as such. This irreversibly leads to inadequate action.

#### *Splitting is a team problem*

The behaviour of victims of sexual abuse (and dealing with it) frequently gives rise to a struggle among the professional caregivers.

This causes splitting phenomena in the healthcare team.[14] In broad terms, the team can be dealt into an 'in-group' and an 'out-group'. This division concerns the perception of the behaviour of the client, the self-image of the professional caregiver and the vision about the necessary support.

1. The perception of the victim of sexual abuse – the professional caregivers who belong to the in-group show understanding for the behavioural escalations and see it as asking for support, predictability and clarity. The out-group experiences the behaviour of the traumatised victim as being demanding and manipulative. They have the feeling of being consciously played off against one another.
2. The self-image of the professional caregiver – the caregivers from the in group feel valued and have a sense of self-confidence. This image is encouraged thanks to the acceptable behaviour of the victim and compliments from parents and colleagues. The caregivers from the out-group mainly have negative experiences with the victim, despite their own efforts. Behavioural escalations frequently occur. This group often feel incapable and become irritated or even emotionally burned out.
3. The vision regarding care and support – the members of the in-group relate the behaviour of the victim to the trauma and advocate support and an adapted individual approach. The caregivers from the out-group look for greater control of the situation and are convinced that there are too few or unclear agreements. They emphasise (group) rules.[15]

The practitioner involved should pay specific attention to the phenomena of splitting during the support of victims of sexual abuse. The spirit of togetherness in the healthcare team can become heavily under pressure and the team can even fall apart, with a destructive effect on the support of victims of sexual abuse.

If the team realises this and is prepared to be open, the phenomena of splitting can be effectively combated. Encouraging open and transparent communication between the team and the healthcare professionals is effective in such situations. The practitioner sets an example here. It is also the task of the practitioner to create a safe environment in which the healthcare professionals' perception of the situation can be discussed. In this way, the team can work together in dealing with the situation of abuse, and isolation of individual healthcare professionals can be prevented.

### 9.1.7 Transference and countertransference

The care and support of a victim of sexual abuse includes the client's personal and intimate feelings. The one-sided openness of the victim can create a 'projection screen'. This means that the victim can project all sorts of illusions, needs, longings and experiences onto the caregiver. This phenomenon is called transference: the victim transfers feelings, fantasies and behaviour which were originally directed towards someone else, onto the caregiver. The actual situation does not match their type or intensity but does, however, play a role. Transference symptoms are not infrequently related to sexuality. The unconditional attention and the understanding of the caregiver helps the victim to feel accepted and valued; this can be confused with falling in love.

In such situations it is possible for the healthcare professional to find themselves in a moment of temptation. Countertransference is the name for the feelings which the client makes the caregiver feel. These can be feelings of falling in love, but also of powerlessness and despair. Unconscious countertransference can have a negative influence on the open attitude and the professional actions of the caregiver. If a caregiver is conscious of countertransference reactions, these can provide important information about the coping process. It is essential that the healthcare team provides a safe environment; this is only possible if a healthcare professional is able to empathise with the client.

#### *Projective identification*

The term 'projective identification' was first used in 1946 by the Austrian/British Melanie Klein, psychologist and founder of the Anglo-Saxon psychoanalysis. Projective identification is a special form of countertransference in which the client subconsciously places certain unmanageable feelings outside themselves and 'lends' them to the caregiver. After abuse, this often concerns feelings regarding sex and aggression. The caregiver should detoxify these unbearable feelings and give them back to the client in a manageable form. In this way, caregiver and client can create a new situation together in which old patterns and experiences can receive new meaning due to the personal reactions of the caregiver. In order to do this and to help the client progress, it is essential that a caregiver is aware of these phenomena and does not react as if the feelings and needs are their own.

The practitioner must discuss the processes of transference and countertransference with the healthcare professionals involved. They should be aware of the cause of the feelings and thoughts of the client, and of the power which these have on the client. Sexual behaviour of a client is a call for protection and not an invitation for sexual contact!

---

It is at all times the task of the healthcare professional to protect the boundaries of intimacy.[16] Peer-to-peer coaching and individual coaching can help in this process of awareness.

---

### 9.1.8 The personal coping process of healthcare professionals

Healthcare professionals are usually focused on looking after others. Looking after themselves usually has the lowest priority. Many healthcare professionals have enormous empathic ability. Due to the way in which they know what a client is feeling, they are able to give the client what they need.

These empathic abilities can, however, get many healthcare professionals into problems. If stress influences their mental and physical health, there is a risk of exhaustion, irritation, desensitisation and sombreness. This can even lead to secondary traumatising. The symptoms of secondary traumatic stress correspond with those of post-traumatic stress. Intrusions, avoidance and increased irritability can occur, as can sleeping problems and loss of concentration (Chapter 4).

Special attention for self-care is essential, definitely in the case of caregivers who work with clients who have been sexually abused. A 'looking after yourself' test[17] and various exercises for self-care are described in Chapter 10.

For healthcare professionals who have suffered sexual abuse (or those in their immediate surroundings), abuse of a client can act as a trigger for all sorts of unprocessed issues. This can make it difficult to support and care for a client (and their system). It is then important to refer the healthcare professional to a course of personal healthcare.

It is also possible that healthcare professionals can use their personal experiences to assist the client and their system.

## 9.2 The SOS programme for healthcare professionals

In the SOS programme we assume that the healthcare professionals involved have already been informed about the (suspected) sexual abuse, according to the protocol. If this is not the case, it is important that the practitioner communicates this news (together with the manager) to the team of healthcare professionals according to the principles of communicating bad news.

Adhering to a (temporary) speaking ban works in a limiting way for those working together and for the coping processes and is for this reason not recommended. It is advised to emphasise the importance of being careful in the way in which information concerning the sexual abuse should be treated. Attention must be paid to a possible police investigation – intensive communication between healthcare professionals and the police is advised at an early stage.

### 9.2.1 Attitude aspects

It is important that the practitioner acts as a role model when discussing difficult subjects and demonstrates resilience and active involvement. The professional should have an open and supportive attitude during the conversations with healthcare professionals. The professional can use (suitable) humour to make sure that the atmosphere does not become too emotionally charged.

The practitioner keeps the healthcare professionals up to date, both inside and outside the sessions. This always takes place (if possible) in agreement with the client and their parents/guardians.

### 9.2.2 Preparation by the professional

For the first session with the healthcare professionals, it is important that the practitioner has done some research into the healthcare professionals involved and the team with which they will be working.

- Is it an experienced team?
- How long have they been working together?
- Have these healthcare professionals been confronted by a (suspicion of) sexual abuse before?

These factors partly determine the effect of the situation on the team and partly influence the choice of content of the sessions and the exercises which will be chosen. Pay attention to the possibility of healthcare professionals having had experience(s) of sexual abuse in their private lives. This also determines the reaction and resilience of the healthcare professional!

It is, of course, also important that the healthcare professionals are kept informed of the content of the sessions with the client and their parents/guardians, so that they can refer to this if required during the daily care for the client.

### 9.2.3 Time and place of the sessions with the healthcare professional

The professional organises four sessions for the healthcare professionals involved. The first session with the healthcare team is held as soon as possible after finding out about the abuse. Depending on the composition of the team, a suitable location is chosen for the session. Make sure that the healthcare professionals can take part in the session without being interrupted and that they have time afterwards to recover and relax before they have to go back to work.

The second session happens about a week later. The third session is a joint session in which the client, their system and the healthcare professionals involved share experiences and learn to communicate with each other about what has happened. This joint session is planned approximately a month after the start of the programme. After eight weeks, a follow-up session is planned for all healthcare professionals involved.

The sessions with the healthcare professionals last for approximately 90 minutes.

### 9.2.4 Separately or together?

The starting point for the healthcare team is that all healthcare professionals involved are present during the sessions. The presence of the manager during the sessions is highly recommended! It can be the case that various healthcare professionals are involved in working with the client who do not usually work together. In that case, it must be considered whether it is best to see the healthcare professionals together or separately.

It may be necessary to speak to healthcare professionals individually. In this case, healthcare professional should be referred for an individual course of support.

### 9.2.5 The structure of the sessions

The sessions for the healthcare professionals are described in this chapter. The order and contents of the issues for the sessions are chosen on the basis of the literature on this subject and on experience. Guidelines are given for the stabilisation of the situation, the inventory of the sexual abuse, emotional support and psychoeducation for the healthcare professionals involved. Alongside practical guidelines for supporting the client, specific attention is also given to the support of the healthcare professionals in their own process and that of their colleagues. Adequate daily support of a client can only take place when the healthcare professionals involved are able to organise and discuss their own experiences and perceptions. The healthcare professional acts as a role model for the client here.

It is important that the professional realises that it is possible to be flexible in conducting the SOS programme, and that this can also be necessary, depending on the situation. Different situations of sexual abuse may require a different emphasis on certain themes, adapted to the incident, the relationship with the perpetrator, the past history, the strengths and weaknesses of the client and their system and the healthcare professionals involved.

---

The SOS programme is not a protocol or straightjacket, but a guideline. The SOS handbook can be added to using personal creativity, and be adapted according to the actual circumstances.

---

### 9.2.6 Using the help book for healthcare professionals

The help book is put together by the practitioner before the first session. In Chapter 10 exercises are described showing ways in which the sexual abuse (and the perception of this) can be discussed, understood and organised with the healthcare professionals involved. The book for healthcare professionals gives space to reconstruct the situation of sexual abuse. The healthcare professional will have the chance to explore and express their own thoughts and feelings about the situation. There is space for describing personal emotions and symptoms and noting questions which arise in between the sessions.

In addition, the importance of the role of the healthcare professional in the victim's coping process after sexual abuse is addressed. There are exercises which focus on the individual healthcare professional as well as those which focus on the team. There is attention given to their own coping process of the healthcare professional and the care for themselves and their colleagues. If necessary, it is possible to put together a help book for the team.

The book for healthcare professionals provides space for the stress reactions of the client. Applicable, practical information is added about making a statement, the studio hearing and dealing with the media. A tab-page for 'other information' is also included so that healthcare professionals can add information to the folder themselves.

## 9.3 The sessions for healthcare professionals

### 9.3.1 Healthcare professionals session 1: as soon as possible

What is needed?

- The SOS handbook

- Help book for healthcare professionals
- Suitable worksheets, for example:
  - 'Talking about sexual abuse' (Chapter 10)
  - 'Thoughts and feelings' (Chapter 10)
  - 'Sexual abuse' (Chapter 10)
  - Safety exercises (Chapter 10).

Duration of the session: 90 minutes.

### *Talking about the sexual abuse with the healthcare professionals involved*

When a client experiences a shocking event, the healthcare professionals involved are often at least as shocked as the client themselves and their systems. It is the task of the practitioner to reconstruct and organise the event together with the healthcare professionals. This leads to more understanding and control of the situation: a requirement for adequate professional action.

The practitioner can reconstruct the event with the professional caregivers involved by using a number of questions:

- When did you find out about the sexual abuse?
- By whom were you told and in which way did you find out about the sexual abuse?
- What did you hear then?
- What was your first thought?
- What feelings does the sexual abuse cause in you as a healthcare professional? (For example: powerlessness, guilt, anger, unsafety, mistrust.)
- What feelings do you have with regard to the (suspected) perpetrator?
- What feelings do you have with regard to the parents of the client(s)?
- What was your first reaction?

- Were these reactions, feelings and thoughts as you would have expected them to be? What surprised you about yourself?
- Have you spoken to someone about this? If you have, then with whom?
- Have you spoken to your colleagues about the situation? If so, describe what you have discussed. If not, why not?
- If applicable, how did your colleague(s) react?
- If applicable, which reactions were as you would have expected them to be? What surprised you about the reactions of your colleagues?
- What effect does this have on you as healthcare team?

The worksheet 'Talking about sexual abuse' (Chapter 10) can be used here. Visual aids can also be used when organising a complex situation. Using drawings, a timeline or genogram is advised in this case.

### *Emotional support for healthcare professionals and team*

For healthcare professionals who work with clients who have been sexually abused, it is essential to share the experiences and seek support from colleagues. Alongside organising the facts concerning the sexual abuse, attention is paid to the perception of the events by the various healthcare professionals. The practitioner should pay specific attention to the similarities and differences between the individual healthcare professionals. What does this imply for the way in which the healthcare team works? Differences should be respected, but obstacles which stand in the way of a common support process can be examined.

This can be done by making an inventory of the concerns and needs on the basis of the following questions:

- What is troubling me as a healthcare professional?
- What is troubling me as a member of the team?
- What do I need in my role as a healthcare professional?
- What do I need in my role as member of the team?

### *Psychoeducation on talking about sexual abuse and stress reactions*

Talking about the sexual abuse requires special attention by the practitioner. Healthcare professionals involved should be aware of how it is essential for an adequate coping process to invite the client to talk about the sexual abuse and their experience of it. For clients who are not able to communicate using language, different forms of expression should be encouraged. Various methods are described in Chapter 7. Also for clients who are able to communicate using language, it is important to use different ways of communication, such as creative or physical activities to stimulate both halves of the brain. Bilateral stimulation has a positive effect on coping with trauma.

Certainly if a statement has already been made with the police, it is important to talk about this properly. To support the caregivers, the information sheet 'Dos and don'ts for talking about sexual abuse with a victim' (Chapter 10) can be handed out and discussed.

Depending on the content of the protocols which are implemented in the healthcare organisations involved, attention should be paid when talking about sexual abuse to minimum fact interviews and the police interview of clients (see Section 3.4.2).

Healthcare professionals need short and concrete guidelines in the *first session* for the support of the client. The practitioner does a quick diagnostic on the basis of the present information (acquired in the client session, but also in the sessions with parents and healthcare professionals involved) about stress reactions of the client. The checklist 'Post-traumatic stress symptoms' can be used here (see Chapter 6).

It is, of course, important to be aware of the behavioural problems which the client displayed before the sexual abuse took place (if this is clear). Observed changes in behaviour are important here. Existing behavioural problems or psychopathology form a risk factor for coping with a shocking event. Support agreements are made with the healthcare team involved, depending on the stress reactions which are observed.

The safety measures which have been taken should be communicated with the healthcare professionals involved. If a police statement is (to be) made, attention should be paid to the support of the client during this process. Here we refer to information about making a statement (or a report) to the police (Section

3.4), supporting the client during this process (Section 3.4.1) and talking with the client about sexual abuse in the context of the police interview (Section.3.4.2).

If a client has to undergo a medical investigation, the healthcare professionals should be informed about this. Here we refer to the information on medical tests (Section 3.5). If the case receives a lot of media attention, it is advised to make agreements at this stage about how to deal with the media (see Chapter 10 and the help book for healthcare professionals).

### *End of the session*

To benefit the support process for the client, caregivers should be aware of the main points of the contents of the sessions with the client and their parents (or significant others). This ensures that they can react to themes and advice which have been discussed. This, of course, happens in agreement with the client and their parents.

If a client lives in a care institution or home, it is important to name a contact person for the parents within the healthcare team, alongside the professional. This makes open and transparent communication easier. It must be clear for all of those involved what the communication plan is: who communicates with whom?

The first session for healthcare professionals ends with information about the book for healthcare professionals and this is handed over. The contents of this book depend on the circumstances and those involved in the situation of abuse. The healthcare professional also has the chance to explore and express their own thoughts and feelings about the situation. If necessary, it is important to name the similarities and differences between the healthcare professionals involved and to make agreements about how these differences can be respected. The book for healthcare professionals provides space for psychoeducation on support needs after sexual abuse and dealing with the client's stress reactions.

For healthcare professionals who have experienced sexual abuse themselves (or in their immediate environment), the abuse can act as a trigger for all sorts of unprocessed issues. It can be difficult to support and care for a client (and their system). It is important that a practitioner highlights this possibility and invites healthcare professionals to talk about it (possibly at a different time). Tell the professional caregivers about the possibility of holding an individual discussion. Provide various possibilities: a talk with the practitioner, manager, confidant or personal relations employee. It may be necessary to refer healthcare professionals for individual help with their own coping process.

It is also possible that healthcare professionals use their personal experiences in order to assist a client and their system in an adequate way.

### 9.3.2 Healthcare professional session 2: after one week

What is needed?

- SOS handbook
- Help book for healthcare professionals
- Appropriate worksheets, for example:
  - 'Dos and don'ts for talking about sexual abuse with a victim' (Chapter 10)
  - 'My fault or not?' (Chapter 10)
  - 'Looking after yourself test' (Chapter 10)
  - Preparation sheet, joint session.

Duration of the session: 90 minutes.

#### *Talking about the sexual abuse with healthcare professionals*

Events are sinking in, or new details may have come to light. Healthcare professionals have spoken to each other, and possibly also with others, about the situation. After a week, the practitioner will talk about what is actually happening, together with the manager concerned. The story will be summed up in short again and possibly added to or adapted. To prevent confusion, transparent communication with the healthcare team involved is advised. The healthcare team should be kept up to date about the possible process of contact with the police. Here attention should be paid to a possible police or legal process.

Safety agreements which have been made are run through again and adjusted where necessary. The communication plan must be clear for all of those involved. Who communicates with whom? The professional tells the healthcare professionals about the main points of the sessions with the clients and their parents. Only information is shared which the client and their parents know is to be shared.

### *Emotional support for the healthcare professionals and team*

Talking about experiences and seeking support from colleagues is essential for healthcare professionals who work with victims of sexual abuse. It is also difficult for healthcare professionals to talk about the perception of a situation of sexual abuse. Feelings of powerlessness, guilt and shame play a role. In the second session, the various healthcare professionals' perceptions of the situation of sexual abuse should be central. The practitioner, preferably together with the manager concerned, should create the opportunity for this. The exercise 'Thoughts and feelings' (Chapter 10) can help to get the conversation going. In the discussion of the thoughts and feelings, special attention should be paid to the similarities and differences between the individual healthcare professionals. What do they mean for the way in which the healthcare team functions? Differences should be respected, but obstacles which stand in the way of a joint support process can also be examined. This can be done by making an inventory of concerns and needs by way of the following questions:

- What is troubling me as a healthcare professional?
- What is troubling me as a member of the team?
- What do I need in my role as a healthcare professional?
- What do I need in my role as member of the team?

### *Psychoeducation on talking about stress symptoms and support needs*

In the second session, specific attention must be paid to the stress symptoms and support needs of the client. According to the available information, the professional makes an estimation of the stress symptoms which play a role for the client(s) concerned and the severity of these. The 'Child/client post-traumatic stress symptoms checklist' can help here (Chapter 10). It is advisable to use the list to let healthcare professionals observe and report about the stress reactions of the client. Agreements about support are made according to the stress symptoms.

The professional provides psychoeducation on the support needs of the client. Themes which are addressed are safety and the perception of safety, reliable care and getting back to normal life. The normal daily routine enhances the feeling of safety, gives the client the feeling of being in control again and lessens anxieties. Encouraging a normal day and night rhythm is essential here.

Positive physical experiences and physical activities should be encouraged. The following information sheets can be used for this purpose: 'How should I react to sexual abuse' (Chapter 10) and 'Dos and don'ts in the support of victims of sexual abuse' (Chapter 10).

In the support of a victim of sexual abuse, a balance must be found between the normal programme and specific attention for the sexual abuse. If a client asks for a lot of attention for their story, it is advised to let contact about the sexual abuse take place at agreed times or to be talked about with agreed people as far as this is possible. The help book for the client can help with this. The professional caregivers must be aware of the contents of the help book, so that they can refer to it if needed during the daily situation. It can also help to agree on a sign with a client, by which they can express that things aren't going well. In this way, the caregiver can respond by offering extra safety or support by distraction or relaxation.

### *End of the session*

At the end of the session it is important to pay attention to the double (and separate) task of the caregiver with regard to their own coping process and in the support for the client and their system.

Tell the professional caregivers about the possibility of holding an individual discussion. Provide various possibilities: a talk with the professional, manager, confidant, human relations employee. It can be necessary to refer healthcare professionals for individual help with their own coping process.

---

Always check whether agreements about safety and communication are clear. This is definitely of great importance in the case of a large client system, multiple clients involved and a lot of media attention.

---

The second session ends with a preparation for the third, joint session with the client, system and (a delegation of) professional caregivers. It is important that caregivers realise that the aim of the session is to support the client together. During this session the client is encouraged to talk about how the people in their environment can help them in the best way.

It is important that the client is excluded from blame by the system: 'It is good that you told others about it. It is not your fault.' The caregivers who are present at the session receive the assignment to think about the positive characteristics and strengths of the client and their system, which can be used in the near future.

Finally, the professional gives a short explanation of the chosen 'Together we are strong' exercise.

### 9.3.3 Joint session: after three weeks

Three weeks after the second session, a joint session is held with the client, the parents/family, the professional caregivers and the practitioner. The session is held in a place which is safe for the client and in the presence of their significant others. The session begins with having something to drink, along with a small snack. This can help to lessen anxiety and restore and enhance mutual relationships.

What is needed?

- SOS handbook
- Help books

- The presence of the manager/team leader as co-leader of the discussion:
    - A small snack to go with the coffee
    - Flip-chart or whiteboard
    - The worksheet 'Together we are strong' (see the help book for the client)
    - Equipment to do the 'Together we are strong' exercise at the end of the discussion, such as drawing and craft supplies. Depending on the client's taste, you can also choose to use glitters and stars, photos, a computer and so on.

After the session you give the help books back. Agree with the professional caregivers how and when they will help the client.

Duration of the session: approximately two hours in total. The joint session lasts for about an hour. Afterwards there is an informal time with everyone involved, with the aim of creating a sense of togetherness, encouraging communication and getting back to normal life.

### The start of the joint session

Tell those involved about the session:

*'We're going to talk together today about what has happened. It is important to do this because everyone is shocked about it. We help each other by talking about it together.'*

Explain clearly how the session will be conducted:

*'We're together here in ...'s room. We'll begin with a cup of coffee or tea and something to eat. I (or someone else, name them here) will lead the session and make sure that the talk goes well. When we've finished talking we'll make something together. When we've finished doing that we'll talk some more together and then we'll finish the session together.'*

### *Talking about the sexual abuse*

The professional, or the manager present, briefly expains what has happened to begin the session. If the police interview has already taken place, it is possible to say more than if the hearing still has to happen. Possibly use a timeline or sociogram to clarify the story.

### *Psychoeducation on stress symptoms and support needs*

Psychoeducation follows, in which the professional explains that everyone involved in the situation is shocked and reacts in their own way:

*'Everyone is very shocked and looks at the situation in their own way. Everyone reacts in their own way. You can be angry, scared or sad. Let's talk about how we have all reacted.'*

It is important that the reactions of parents and healthcare professionals are prepared during their own sessions. The joint session is intended as support for the client. Parents and professional caregivers can describe their reaction in short and emphasise that the client has done well to tell what is bothering them. Then parents and caregivers can explain that what has happened was not the client's fault. The can also explicitly say that it is not the client's fault that they are now feeling sad.

Positive strengths and characteristics of the client should be mentioned, such as how well the client is coping, despite the bad things that have happened; for example, 'I was angry/scared'. Then tell the client, *'You did well to tell about it (if this is how it came to light) and you are dealing with it well. It is not your fault that I feel like this now. It is the perpetrator's fault. They were wrong. Not you.'*

It is important to direct the contents of the discussion in this direction and (if necessary) to add this information yourself. Clients must be empowered and excluded from blame! Any necessary support for other participants in the session must be referred to a different time.

### *Together we are strong!*

The client is asked how they are feeling now and what they have to say. The person who led session 2 helps the client to describe what is bothering them. Attention is paid to practical issues, safety and reactions to what parents and healthcare professionals have said. There is also space for the wishes of the client with regard to the near future.

How can the client be helped in the best way and what do they need help with? What does the client like and what helps?

The 'Together we are strong' exercise is meant to break through the isolation that people experience after a disturbing event. The aim is to let the client experience that everyone is working together and helping to make the abuse 'bearable'.

The professional introduces a suitable 'Together we are strong' exercise in the help book of the client and explains, in a way that is adapted to the client, that the abuse hurts. Suitable exercises are, for example:

- 'Together we are strong – the plaster' (Section 6.3)
- 'Together we are strong – the message' (Section 6.3)
- 'Together we are strong – the song' (Section 6.3)
- 'Together we are strong – music' (Section 7.4).

### *End of the session – evaluation talk: what did we think of this discussion?*

The session ends by asking those involved what they thought of the session. You can choose to do this together or individually with the client. This choice depends on how the talk goes, the characteristics of the parents (are there also parent issues, are emotions heavily charged?) and of the client (can he/she cope with evaluating the session together or would it be better to do this in a separate place?).

Write about the talk in the client's help book (or let the client write themselves) about the talk and what they thought about it. Put the joint exercise, or a photo of it, in the help book as well and give it to the client to take home with them.

### *What next?*

Agree and write down who the client will receive support from in the following weeks and at which moments. Say that they will support the client now and that the client doesn't have to visit you for the next few weeks. Say that you will make an appointment in two months to see how everyone is feeling and how help will be provided. Make concrete agreements and write these down in the help books of those involved.

Then a link will be made back to the client's life, for example by talking with those involved about the rest of the day.

### 9.3.4 Healthcare professional session 3: follow-up – after two months

What is needed?

- SOS handbook
- Help book for parents
- Suitable worksheets, for example:
  - 'Secondary traumatic stress checklist' (Chapter 10)
  - 'Support from people around you' (Chapter 10)
  - 'SOS evaluation form' (Chapter 10).

Duration of the session: 90 minutes.

#### *Talking about the sexual abuse*

After two months the professional evaluates the process together with the manager concerned: which safety measures have been taken, who has been informed, how is the contact with the police? There is attention for the perceptions of the healthcare professionals (powerlessness, guilt, anger) and the symptoms and support of the client.

#### *Psychoeducation on secondary traumatising*

It is important for the practitioner to provide psychoeducation on secondary traumatising (Chapter 10). Healthcare professionals can be affected by classic symptoms of PTSD due to the confrontation with traumatised clients. These can include disturbing thoughts and fantasies which are associated with the traumatic experiences of clients, nightmares, anxieties and overly startled reactions in everyday situations. This can lead to an increase in feelings of alienation and isolation, in both working life and in private life. Providing help to people who are seriously psychologically damaged can lead to a burn-out in the healthcare professional. Symptoms of this are apathy, getting tired quickly, heaviness of mood, forgetfulness, isolation, irritability and headache. These are symptoms of emotional exhaustion, which occur gradually.

Paying frequent and adequate attention to the perception of healthcare professionals who are working with traumatised clients lessens the risk of secondary traumatising and burn-out. If secondary traumatising or burn-out is indicated, however, personal healthcare treatment is then required for the healthcare professional.

### *Emotional support for individual healthcare professionals and the team*

Many healthcare professionals have the tendency to forget about their own needs and to concentrate on looking after others. Personal needs are ignored in an attempt to be a good healthcare professional. It is important to remember that looking after ourselves is essential, particularly in the case of those who work with clients who have been sexually abused.

---

Only when we look after ourselves well will we be able to look after the client properly. In this way we can act as a positive role model for the client, who often doesn't look after themselves well.

---

A self-care test is described in Chapter 10, which healthcare professionals can fill in to check whether they are looking after themselves properly (Looking after yourself test). In the test, questions are asked about: a little or a lot of sleep, nightmares, too little, too much or unhealthy eating, excessive use of alcohol or drugs and coffee, feelings of being numbed, startled reactions, isolation behaviour, sombreness, forgetfulness, irritability and physical symptoms. If necessary, the healthcare professional – independently or with support – can make a personal self-care plan.

For healthcare professionals who have experienced sexual abuse themselves, or in their immediate environment, the abuse of the client can act as a trigger for all sorts of unprocessed issues from the past. This can make it difficult to support and care for the client and their system. In such situations, it is important to refer a healthcare professional for personal healthcare treatment. Always state the possibility of an individual talk for caregivers. Offer various possibilities: a talk with the professional, manager, confidant or human relations employee.

It is also possible that healthcare professionals can use their personal experiences to assist the client and their system in an adequate way.

### *End of the session and evaluation*

At the end of the session it is important to pay attention to the process of coping with trauma. Eighty per cent of the people who have experienced a single trauma and are supported in a beneficial way by those around them recover on the basis of their own resilience. This percentage is lower for people with an intellectual disability and for people who have been traumatised for a long period of time.

Healthcare professionals must be aware of the fact that once a person has been a victim of sexual abuse, they run a greater risk of becoming a victim again, particularly if the client demonstrates sexually solicitous behaviour. This requires much supervision of the client.

Finally, the SOS programme can be evaluated by the healthcare professionals with the help of the SOS evaluation form (Chapter 10). What did they think of the help offered? What do they still need to be able to deal with the situation well?

## SUMMARY

Central to this chapter is the first aid support for healthcare professionals who are involved in working with a client who has become a victim of sexual abuse. During the sessions there is special attention given to the support of the healthcare professionals in their own coping process and that of their colleagues. Adequate daily care and support of a client is only possible if the healthcare professionals involved are able to organise and discuss their own experiences and perceptions. The healthcare professional acts as role model for the client. Guidelines are given for stabilising the situation, making an inventory of the sexual abuse, providing emotional support and psychoeducation for the healthcare professionals involved.

Guidelines are provided for caring for a client who has been made victim of sexual abuse. This emphatically concerns the support – not the treatment! – of victims (and their system) in their daily living environment.

Chapter 10

# EXERCISES FOR THE SUPPORT OF PARENTS, CAREGIVERS AND PROFESSIONAL CAREGIVERS

## Introduction

During the SOS sessions, the professional discusses many issues with the parents and professional caregivers. Various exercises are described in this chapter, which can be helpful in talking about these issues. The exercises are divided into seven trauma-related themes: safety, worries, hurt, fear, anger, relaxation and survival. These exercises are combined in a help book for parents and caregivers. This help book is put together before the first conversation and added to during each session.

The contents of the help book and the choice of exercises and information sheets depends on the individual situation of the parents or team of healthcare professionals. There is no fixed list of contents for the help book; this would not do justice to the diverse situations that one encounters in real life.

In agreement with the parents, the professional selects which worksheets are appropriate for the parents/relatives concerned and at which time they should be used.

To make the help book, the professional can use a folder with various tab-pages. The help book consists of the tab pages: first session, second session, joint session and fourth session. A standard worksheet is provided for the preparation and evaluation of the sessions. The information sheets provide background information for the parents and professional caregivers about the issues which are covered. These information sheets can be added to the help book, if and when the subjects have been discussed during the session. A tab-page 'letters and forms' is also included so that parents can add correspondence and other forms and letters to the folder themselves.

The professional gives the parents and healthcare professionals the following instructions about using the help book:

*'This help book is for you. You can use it to collect and store information about the abuse. There are various tab-pages in the folder. Behind these tab-pages you will see a number of forms which you can fill in during the sessions. There are, for example, forms on which you can write your own thoughts and feelings about the abuse. You can also keep a note here of feelings and questions which arise in between the sessions and which are important to talk about together.*

*'There is also a page on which you can both keep a note of your own symptoms. This may seem exaggerated, but it does prove to be useful. The strange thing about symptoms is that, when you have had them for a long period of time, you can get used to them and don't really notice them anymore. And we want to know how your symptoms are and if they are changing. That's why it's good to keep a note of them. It is, of course, not compulsory to fill in the form, but I do recommend it.*

*'I will also give you information about issues which we have discussed together and so you will be able to read this through in your own time. You can keep these information sheets in this folder and maybe add to them with information from the internet, or information you have received from other people.*

*'Behind the tab-page "letters and forms", you can, for example, keep letters and forms about the police statement and information from the police.'*

# General information and psychoeducation exercises

## Information sheet: Sexual abuse

### What is sexual abuse?

Sexual abuse is a complex issue. It can vary between being forced to endure sexual acts, perform sexual acts on others or perform sexual acts yourself. It can involve watching others perform sexual acts or watching pornographic material which is not suitable for the age or developmental level of the victim.

In every form of sexual abuse there is a power difference between perpetrator and victim. This can be due to a difference in age, developmental level, physical strength or social position, or due to a relationship of dependence. Perpetrators sometimes use a less subtle form of force, such as threats of violence, emotional or psychological pressure or blackmail in order to force the victim to perform sexual acts and keep them secret.

Sexual contact between a person without an intellectual disability and a person with an intellectual disability is not by definition sexual abuse. We assume that people with an intellectual disability have the right to their own sexuality and sexual experiences and that they may make their own choice about this.[1] The requirement is that they are able to give their consent concerning the sexual contact. The concept of 'consent' is important in understanding sexual violence in people with an intellectual disability. In definitions of sexual violence in people with an intellectual disability, alongside the concept of not 'wanting' it, the concept of 'not being able to give consent' is therefore also added.

### Who is sexually abused?

Everyone can be confronted by sexual abuse, regardless of age, place of origin and so on. It happens to girls, boys, women and men across the

1 Bewerking van werkvorm uit: Groenbos, S., Hout, A. and Zon, C. van der (1996) *Omgaan met een seksueel misbruikt kindeen cursus voor pleegouders*. Amsterdam: Federatie Pleegzorg, Hogeschool van Amsterdam, Stichting Therapeutische Gezinsverpleging.

whole world. People with an intellectual disability run a considerably higher risk of being made a victim of sexual abuse as a result of an accumulation of factors.[2] This is mainly caused by the fact that nearly all abuse takes place in relationships of dependence and that people with an intellectual disability remain in these relationships more often and for a longer period of time than others.

## Why do people not tell others straightaway about sexual abuse?

People can have various reasons not to tell others that they are being sexually abused. They can, for example, be afraid of the reactions after disclosure, have feelings of shame and guilt, or be afraid that they will not be believed, with all the associated consequences. If the perpetrator is well known to the victim, then the victim can be worried about this person getting into trouble. The victim can also be concerned about the pain and sadness which the disclosure would bring to significant others in their life. People with an intellectual disability often do not tell others about the abuse because they do not know who they could tell about it. They are often not able to comprehend the incidents and, due to a limited understanding of cause and effect, do not know to what extent they themselves are guilty of what has happened. Perpetrators often play on this confusion by emphasising that the client also enjoys it. It is also possible that the perpetrator forces the client to keep it a secret, for example by using or threatening violence against the victim or their close family.

## What can you do if someone tells you about sexual abuse?

If somebody tells you about sexual abuse, it is important to remain calm and to listen properly. Avoid discussions, do not interrupt or try to play 'detective'; do not ask questions such as who, what and where. Compliment the person for telling you about the abuse, assure them that they are not guilty of what has happened, and arrange help.

## What is important in coping with sexual abuse?

Safety is an important concept in coping with sexual abuse. It must be ensured that the victim feels safe, in both physical and emotional terms. The amount of emotional and social support which a person receives after experiencing sexual abuse, and the extent to which people react in an appropriate way to the abuse, are of great influence in the coping process.

---

2 Berlo, W. van *et al.* (2011) *Beperkt weerbaareen onderzoek naar seksueel geweld bij mensen met een lichamelijke, zintuiglijke of verstandelijke beperking*. Utrecht: Rutgers WPF/Movisie.

# Information sheet: Facts and fables about sexual abuse

**Fable:** Sexual abuse seldom happens.

**Fact:** International research indicates that sexual abuse occurs frequently.[1, 2, 3, 4] Results of research in the Netherlands state that 39 per cent of women and 7 per cent of men without an intellectual disability have been victimised by sexual violence. The percentage of men and women who have been raped is estimated at 10 per cent and 1 per cent respectively.[5]

People with an intellectual disability form a more vulnerable group regarding the risk of sexual abuse and maltreatment. In international literature, it is stated that people with an intellectual disability are three to five times more often the victim of sexual abuse than others in society.[6, 7, 8, 9, 10, 11]

Research in the Netherlands also concludes that people with an intellectual disability run a higher risk of experiencing sexual abuse. Results from the research 'Limitedly resilient' from van Berlo and

---

1 Rozee, P. and Koss, M. (2001) 'Rape: a century of resistance.' *Psychology of Women Quarterly*, 25, 295–311.

2 Garcia-Moreno, C., Jansen, H., Ellsberg, M., Heise, L. and Watts, C. (2005) WHO *Multi-Country Study on Women's Health and Domestic Violence Against Women*. Geneva: WHO Library Catalogen.

3 Johnson, H., Ollus, N. and Nevala, S. (2008) *Violence Against Women: An International Perspective*. New York: Springer.

4 Lalor, K. and McElvaney, R. (2010) 'Child sexual abuse, links to later sexual exploitation/high risk sexual behaviour and prevention/treatment programs.' *Trauma, Violence & Abuse*, 11 (4), 159–177.

5 Bakker, F., Graaf, H. de, Haas, S. de, Kedde, H., Kruijer, H. and Wijsen, C. (2009) *Seksuele gezondheid in Nederland*. Utrecht: Rutgers Nisso groep.

6 Baladarian, N. (1991) 'Sexual abuse of people with developmental disabilities.' *Journal of Sexuality and Disability*, 9 (4), 323–335.

7 Sobsey, D. and Doe, T. (1991) 'Patterns of sexual abuse and assault.' *Sexuality and Disability*, 9 (3), 243–259.

8 Gorman-Smith, D. and Matson, J. L. (1992) 'Sexual Abuse and Persons with Developmental Disabilities.' In W. T. O'Donohue and A. Geer (eds) *The Sexual Abuse of Children: Theory, Research, and Therapy*. Hillsdale, NJ: Lawrence-Erlbaum Association.

9 Westat Inc. (1991/1993) *A Report on the Maltreatment of Children with Disabilities*. Washington DC: US Department of Health and Human Services.

10 Gordon, B. N. and Schroeder, C. S. (1995) *Sexuality: A Developmental Approach to Problems*. New York: Plenum Publishing Corp.

11 Hingsberger, D. and Melberg Schwier, K. (2000) *Sexuality, Your Sons and Daughters with Intellectual Disabilities*. London: Jessica Kingsley Publishers.

colleagues states that 61 per cent of women and 23 per cent of men with an intellectual disability have experienced sexual violence in their lives. The sexual violence which they report varies from being touched in a harmful way, to rape. Rape is reported by 23 per cent of women and 7 per cent of men with an intellectual disability.[12]

It is stated in various publications that 40 per cent of people with an intellectual disability become victim of abuse and/or mistreatment before the age of 18.[13]

**Fact:** Sexual abuse occurs in most cases by someone who is known and trusted. About 90 per cent of reported sexual abuse is perpetrated by a family member or well-known acquaintance. International research reveals that in 25 per cent of cases of sexual abuse of people with an intellectual disability, the perpetrator is an employee of a care organisation.[14]

The fact that a person is dependent on a professional healthcare worker increases the risk of sexual abuse.

**Fable:** You should not inform young children about sexual abuse, this will only make them fearful.

**Fact:** Talking with young children about the body parts where they are allowed to be touched and the parts where they are not allowed to be touched has a helpful effect rather than a frightening effect.

**Fable:** People who have experienced sexual abuse never get over it.

**Fact:** With good psychological first aid, support from those around them and possible additional trauma treatment, people are able to cope with life after sexual abuse.

**Fable:** Talking about sexual abuse only makes it worse for the victim.

---

12 Berlo *et al*. 2011.
13 Commissie Samson (2012) *Omringd door zorg, toch niet veilig. Seksueel misbruik van door de overheid uit huis geplaatste kinderen, 1945-heden*. Amsterdam: Boom.
14 Sobsey and Doe 1991.

**Fact:** Talking about sexual abuse gives the victim the opportunity to express their feelings and fears and has a healing effect.

**Fable:** Boys who have been abused will later become homosexual.

**Fact:** A connection has never been found between sexual abuse and homosexuality. However, boys who have been made victim by male perpetrators can doubt their own sexual preference due to having had feelings of sexual excitement during the abuse.

**Fable:** Boys who have been sexually abused later become perpetrators themselves.

**Fact:** If a boy receives good help after the disclosure of abuse, including psychological first aid and possibly also treatment, then there is generally not an increased chance of him becoming a perpetrator himself in comparison with other boys. The chance of the risk increasing depends more on the boy's past history than on his personality.

# Information sheet: How should I react to sexual abuse?

- Make sure that you are calm.
- Do not be scared to talk about it.
- Find a place where you will not be disturbed.
- Try to listen well, avoid discussions and answer questions.
- Accept possible strong reactions from the client/child.
- Agree with the client/child where, and at which times, they can talk to you.
- Agree on a sign, which the client can use to express that they want to talk to you.
- Avoid negative and trivialising reactions about the abuse, such as, 'How could you have been so stupid?', 'Why didn't you walk away, or push him away from you?'
- Avoid well-meant advice such as, 'Don't think about it anymore', 'Try to forget about it'.
- Make agreements about whom the client wants to talk to about the events, in the house, in the family and at school.
- Always give correct and direct information.
- Try to control your own emotions in the presence of the client/child.
- Pay attention to verbal and non-verbal signs from the client/child.
- Praise the client/child extensively if they have told you about it themselves.
- Say that you care about the client/child and will help them as much as possible: we'll get you through this together!
- Give the client/child positive attention.
- Express that it is not the client/child's fault and keep repeating this.

- Be aware of the emotions of the client/child.
- Do not express threats to the perpetrator in the presence of the child/client. This increases the client/child's fear.
- Keep to the boundaries which you normally apply.
- Also pay attention to the brothers and sisters or other clients: they can also think that it is their own fault. Say that it is not the brother/sister/other client's fault.
- Explain to family and friends that children who are sexually abused can panic about physical contact which they have not initiated themselves.
- If people tell you that they would know what they would do if they were in your shoes, then explain that they are not actually in your shoes and that their comments do not help. Explain what you do want (love, attention, to cry and so on).

# Information sheet: Dos and don'ts for talking about sexual abuse with a victim

| Dos | Don'ts |
|---|---|
| Create opportunities for talking about the sexual abuse. | Avoid the subject of sexual abuse. Keep trying to get the story out of an avoidant person who is showing much resistance. |
| Encourage the expression of feelings and thoughts about the sexual abuse by talking, playing, movement or creative activities. | Say that a client mustn't think about it or has to forget it. |
| Stay calm and aware if the client tells you something about the abuse and try to write down as precisely as possible what the client has told you. | Panic and be surprised, sad or angry. |
| If the client's story falters for a while, show your interest by nodding or making interested sounds. | Interrupt the client when they are telling you about the sexual abuse. |
| Ask open questions, which begin with question words such as who, what and where: 'What happened then?', 'Can you tell me some more about it?' | Ask closed and suggestive questions, such as, 'Did he also touch your breasts?' |
| Tell the client who is going to be told about the story in order to make adequate action possible. | Promise to keep it secret – keeping it a secret makes adequate support for a victim impossible. |
| Tell the client/child which steps will be taken; be open about this. Remain brief and to the point. Do not bother the client/child with all sorts of procedure details. | Bother the client/child with practical matters concerning the abuse – protect them from this. |
| These guidelines must be adapted for the individual client. This should happen in consultation with a professional. | Tell half-truths! |

# Information sheet: Reactions to trauma

The reactions which occur in people who have experienced a shocking event can be divided into three categories. The stress reactions described here are normal reactions to extreme events. They will generally fade after a few weeks and eventually disappear.

## Avoidance or becoming withdrawn

In the case of avoidance or becoming withdrawn, people try to avoid all memories of the traumatic event. They do not want to talk about it, avoid places, things or people which remind them of the incident, or deny that it has happened. People can also lose interest in certain hobbies, or have the feeling that they are numbed and cut off from their normal life. This emotional flatness can cause feelings of estrangement and loneliness, with negative thoughts about the future. Avoidance can occur both consciously and subconsciously.

## Increased irritability

Increased irritability is expressed by being exaggeratedly alert and jumpy, as if being constantly wary of new danger. They are exaggeratedly on the look-out and are startled quickly. People can have difficulty concentrating, difficulty with falling asleep or staying asleep, or become angry or frightened quickly.

## Intrusions

An intrusion means that a person re-experiences the traumatic experience through repetitive and profoundly unpleasant memories of the incident. These images and memories invade the mind during peaceful situations or when the person is alone. People can react in intense ways, both physically and emotionally, to things which remind them of the traumatic experience. This can include sounds, scents, tastes, places, people; these are referred to as 'trauma reminders'. Nightmares can occur about the traumatic incident. Traumatised children can often be troubled by frightening dreams without recognisable content. Another specific re-experiencing reaction in children is post-traumatic play.

# Information sheet: Overview reactions and needs of the child/client

| Reactions of the child/client | Need of the child/client |
|---|---|
| Fear. | Safety, protection, recognition, patience, simplifying of tasks. |
| Guilt. | Reassurance. |
| Constantly scared that something is going to happen. | Structure, consistency, facts, information, simplifying tasks. |
| Being exaggeratedly alert. | |
| Helplessness. | Physical care, simplifying tasks and expectations. |
| Chaotic: losing control of feelings and emotions. | Peacefulness, a calm environment. |
| Tiredness. | Sleep, predictability, peace and quiet. |
| Constantly retelling the story or acting it out. | Somebody who listens. |
| Fear of being alone, having difficulty with saying goodbye to other people. | Safety, clarity about where the other person is going and when they will be back; reassurance that the person will be safe. |
| Confusion, forgetfulness, concentration, problems. | Simplifying tasks, repetition, structure, patience, saying that concentration problems can be an after-effect of trauma. |
| Worrying about something else happening to them. | Reassurance, increasing the feeling of safety. |

# Information sheet: Dos and don'ts in the support of victims of sexual abuse

| Dos | Don'ts |
|---|---|
| Take measures to ensure safety; do this in collaboration with all environments which the child/client visits. | Try to cut the child off from the 'big bad world'. |
| Give the victim a feeling of safety by being directive.<br>Give the victim control over the situation by limited choice possibilities. | Take over all decision making for the victim to unburden them. |
| Try to keep as much as possible to normal daily routines. | Let the child/client stay at home without daytime activities. |
| Be open and reliable; do what you say and say what you do. | Hide the truth in order to protect the victim. |
| React in an understanding and accepting way to stress reactions.<br>Use 'time-in' to provide safety and offer alternative behaviour. | Use time-out as punishment. |
| Reduce external sources of stress such as the internet, social media and TV. | Let the child/client watch TV or use the internet and social media unattended. |
| Ensure positive physical experiences by relaxation, body care and physical exercise. | Let the child/client lie in bed all day long, or hang around on the sofa. |
| Offer consolation in a way that suits the relationship you have with the client. | Offer the client physical closeness without boundaries. |
| Take physical symptoms seriously: in consultation with the professional and/or doctor. | Trivialise physical symptoms. |
| Ensure reinstatement of normal life: if and when safe, get back to school and work. | Show no understanding for the changeable functioning of the child/client after a shocking incident. |
| These guidelines should of course be adapted to the individual client. Safety, and an approach which suits the developmental age of the child/client, must be the guiding factors! Guidelines should only be followed on consultation with a professional. | Show no understanding for a temporary reduction of skills. |

# Information sheet: Reporting and making a statement of sexual abuse

**What is a report of sexual abuse?**
A report of sexual abuse means nothing other than letting the police know about what has happened to you or telling them about something you know has happened. The police will regard this as information and shall in principle not take further action themselves.

**What is official prosecution?**
It is different in the case of the incident being so serious that the police have to get involved immediately, for example if the abuse is still taking place. The judicial authorities can then decide to officially prosecute a criminal offence. The police can authorise an investigation without a statement having been made.

**Can the police do anything with a report?**
A report is usually filed in the police computer system, so that it can always be found again at a later date.

**Will the police talk to the person who has been accused by the person filing the report, when asked to do so by that person, without a statement having been made?**
This is highly uncommon. There is no legal foundation to speak to someone about their behaviour, without an investigation being conducted by the police or judicial authorities. The accused person would then be labelled as a suspect or perpetrator merely on the grounds of a report.

**What is a statement?**
A statement is information which is given to the police stating that a criminal offence has occurred, in which the person who makes the statement asks for the criminal offence to be investigated and the judicial authorities are asked to prosecute. A police statement consists of an official report, in which the declarant states all they know about the criminal offence. The declarant and the police sign the official report. Then the statement becomes a fact and the police can begin the investigation.

**I do not know if I want to make a statement, but I do want more information, is that possible?**
You can always visit the vice department for an informative conversation. After that you can decide what you wish to do. Make an appointment (by

telephone) beforehand. If you have many questions, then make a note of these so that you do not forget to ask any questions. An informative conversation does not make it compulsory to make a statement.

**What happens after making a statement?**

The police investigation starts after the statement has been made. The police investigator begins the search for evidence. Co-operation of the victim can be requested for this aim. If an investigation is experienced as being too overwhelming, the victim is allowed to refuse to work together with the police. If the victim wishes, they can be kept informed on the progress of the investigation. It can, however, be the case that the police do not give any information for a long time after the statement has been made. This does not in any way mean that the police are not doing anything with the statement.

If you as victim wish to know more about how the investigation is going, then you can ask the police investigator who is handling the case about how the case is progressing. It is possible that the investigator cannot complete the investigation, for example because the perpetrator cannot be found or if there is insufficient evidence. It is then probable that the police will decide to let the case rest. This does not mean that the police do not believe the victim. The police basically assume that the story is true, but they cannot provide any, or enough, juridical evidence to prove it. In such situations, a court case will not be held. If the victim has a different opinion about this, he or she can make this known to the investigator concerned, their superior or in exceptional circumstances, to the public prosecutor.

When the police investigator has completed the investigation and found sufficient evidence against the suspect, the dossier is then sent to the public prosecutor.

**When to make a statement**

Making a statement as soon as possible is of great importance for a police investigation, certainly if the offence took place recently. It is then possible that traces are still present. You can, of course, also make a statement if the abuse took place a long time ago. If you want to know whether you can make a statement in your situation, you can ask the police about this.

# Information sheet: Studio hearing

In the case of sexual abuse concerning children under 18 years old, people with an intellectual disability or people with a cognitive affective syndrome, the police interview is conducted by specially trained police agents, in a studio hearing. The hearing then takes place in a special audio visual studio.[1]This studio is furnished in a child-friendly way and provides the opportunity of making a video of the hearing.

Together with those involved, it is considered whether or not the child/person with a disability has to talk to the police or whether this will take place in the special studio. As a rule, the parents/carers of the child and the public prosecutor have to give permission for the hearing. It is also carefully noted who may watch the recording, how this is kept and when it will be deleted.

Given the complexity of such hearings, external experts who are specialised in questioning people with an intellectual disability, play an important advisory role. In the preparation stage these people can, for example, give advice about the best way to communicate with the person concerned and about the plan for the hearing. The external expert can also give advice from the central control room during the hearing. In exceptional cases, on request by the criminal investigator and the public prosecutor, an external expert can also be present during the hearing,

If serious problems are encountered when questioning a person with an intellectual disability, it is possible – on authorisation from the public prosecutor – for the external expert to question the person themselves. This occurs in cases involving people with multiple disabilities or, for example, people with an intellectual disability who need to be questioned by using pictograms.

If there is a difference of opinion between the external expert and the criminal investigator regarding the questioning of a person with an intellectual disability, then the public prosecutor will make the final decision.

Before the hearing takes place in a studio, the child/person with an intellectual disability and, if possible, also the parents and professional caregivers, will be well prepared for the hearing. They can take a look in the studio and the central control room. It is explained to them that recordings will be made of the conversation.

---

1 Openbaar Ministerie (2011) Aanwijzing opsporing en vervolging inzake seksueel misbruik.

When the hearing in the studio has finished, the child/person with an intellectual disability and the parents/professional caregivers are informed of what has happened. During this conversation, if and when necessary, advice is given about possible help or support for the child/client.

The conversations which the police conduct in the audio visual studio are intended for use in legal proceedings and are therefore not of a therapeutic or diagnostic nature.

Recording a conversation in the audio visual studio has a number of advantages. There is a lesser chance that later in the investigation it will be necessary to talk to the child/person with an intellectual disability again. Sometimes a child or person with an intellectual disability will find it difficult to talk about something and would prefer to act it out. This is possible during the hearing in the audio visual studio as it can be watched again on video. In this way, the child/person with an intellectual disability can clearly express the behaviour, movements and facial expressions in a non-verbal way.

Finally, the video recording makes it possible to assess whether the police officer has influenced the hearing, or an expert can be asked to give their opinion, upon request by the judge.

# Information sheet: Dealing with the media

When a suspicion of sexual abuse becomes known, particularly if people with an intellectual disability are involved, large media interest can suddenly occur. What is important if this happens?

- Operate in a proactive way as a care organisation and portray an attitude of openness and transparency.
- Inform parents, relatives and others involved before media reports take place.
- Write a clear press report instead of refusing to provide information.
- Appoint one spokesperson within the organisation.
- Ensure that all employees know the name of this spokesperson, so that they can refer people to them when people from the press contact the organisation.
- Employees, other than the spokesperson, should be instructed in a positive and friendly manner to refrain from giving comments.
- The client and their social system must be prepared for (sudden) contact with the media or information appearing on social media.
- Others clients and parents must be prepared for (sudden) contact with the media or information appearing on social media.

# Information sheet: Tips for and from parents[1]

- Make sure that the police are aware of the developmental level of your child.
- As parents, request that the questioning of your child is done by someone who has been specially educated to question people with an intellectual disability.
- Always ask the police for copies of the witness statements immediately.
- Demand from the care organisation that the victim and (suspected) perpetrator are kept apart.
- Ask for an insight into the plan of action for your child in the short and long term. (The inspectors of care organisations make it compulsory to have these plans.)
- If the incident is due to negligence, carelessness, lack of staff, insufficient supervision, cost savings and so on then seek a lawyer with experience in these cases and hold the organisation responsible.
- Do not let yourself be influenced or intimidated by the care organisation.
- Do not be talked into only making a complaint without making a statement. A complaint is often internally processed within the care organisation and that often takes a very long time.
- From the start, ask for reports of all conversations/meetings which are conducted within the care organisation as a result of the incident.
- If it does actually take a long time, seek publicity.
- Be prepared for a lonely struggle: after a short period of sympathy everyone else will get back to normal life, while you will not yet be ready to do so.
- Make sure that you don't fall into social isolation: take initiatives by making contact if others find it difficult to do so.
- See if you can also get help yourself, for example psychological support via your general practitioner.
- Look after yourself and each other as partners!

1 Freely adapted from L. and E. de Jong.

# Worksheet: Talking about sexual abuse

| **Name:** | |
|---|---|
| Describe how you found out about the sexual abuse (by whom, how and when were you told?) | |
| What was your first thought about it? | |
| Which feelings does the sexual abuse raise in you? (powerlessness, guilt, anger, unsafety, distrust) | |
| What was your first reaction? | |
| Which feelings do you have towards the (suspected) perpetrator? | |
| Were these reactions, feelings and thoughts as you had expected them to be? | |
| What surprised you about yourself? | |
| Have you spoken to anyone about it? | |
| Have you spoken to family members/ friends/ acquaintances about it? If so, describe what you said to whom. | |
| How did they react? | |
| What went as expected? | |
| What surprised you about the reactions of family members/friends/ acquaintances? | |
| What does it do to you as a family/ team? | |
| Which questions do you still have? | |

# Worksheet: Secondary traumatic stress checklist

| | Yes | No |
|---|---|---|
| I am startled more quickly now than I was before. | | |
| I'm scared that something is going to happen to my children or loved ones. | | |
| I have difficulty concentrating. | | |
| I see images in my mind of the shocking incident at unexpected moments. | | |
| I don't sleep well. | | |
| In my spare time I don't want to be confronted by violence anymore; in the news, television programmes or films, for example. | | |
| I can't listen to complicated stories at home or at work. | | |
| I feel tired and exhausted. | | |
| I'm quickly irritated at home and at work. | | |
| I have become distrustful of other people. | | |

## Worksheet: Stress symptoms

Please fill in the table with all the symptoms that you are experiencing or have experienced.

| Date | Symptom | Description |
|---|---|---|
| | | |
| | | |
| | | |
| | | |
| | | |

# Worksheet: Looking after yourself test

How often do you eat breakfast?

1. Nearly every day
2. Once or twice a week
3. Every month
4. What is breakfast?

When did you last have a good laugh?

1. A few days ago
2. Last week
3. Last month
4. In 1972

How often do you spend time with a friend or with friends?

1. Nearly every day
2. Once or twice a week
3. Every month
4. When I see someone at the shops

How often do you have contact with other educators/caregivers?

1. Nearly every day
2. Once or twice a week
3. Every month
4. Hardly ever

How often do you watch a film or television programme which you really want to see?

1. Nearly every day
2. Once or twice a week
3. Every month
4. I can't remember the last time

When did you last say 'no' to something which you really didn't want to do (or which you didn't feel that you were able to do)?

1. This morning
2. Last week
3. Last month
4. I have never even thought of doing this

When was the last time that someone looked after you?

1. Yesterday
2. Last week
3. This year sometime
4. 1973

How often do you sleep enough in order to feel rested the next day?

1. Most nights
2. Once or twice a week
3. Once every month
4. I'm too tired to remember

When did you last read something for your own enjoyment?

1. Today
2. Last week
3. Last month
4. In the third year of secondary school

How often do you meditate or pray?

1. Nearly every day
2. Once or twice a week
3. Once every month
4. Never

How often do you take time to be sexy?

1. Nearly every day
2. Once or twice a week
3. Once a month
4. What is sexy?

How often do you do sports or something physical?

1. Nearly every day
2. Once or twice a week
3. Once every month
4. Does doing the housework count?

## Scores:

Answer 1: 3 points
Answer 2: 2 points
Answer 3: 1 point
Answer 4: 0 points

Add up the points you scored.

**36–24 points:** Congratulations, you have found a good balance between looking after yourself and looking after others. Keep this up!

**23–12 points:** You are definitely doing things to meet your own needs, but you can do more to look after yourself better.

**Less than 12 points:** It looks as if you do too much for others and too little for yourself. Think about your own needs!

This 'looking after yourself test' is based on Coppens and van Kregten's work.[1]

1 Coppens, L. and Kregten, C. van (2012) *Zorgen voor getraumatiseerde kinderen: een training voor opvoeders. Handboek voor trainers*. Houten: Bohn Stafleu van Loghum.

# Worksheet: Child/client post-traumatic stress symptoms checklist

Intrusions

- intrusive unpleasant memories (thoughts and images)
- re-living the sexual abuse (perception and play)
- fearful dreams
- psychological upset at triggers which are related to the abuse.

Avoidance

- avoiding specific things, places or people
- distorting the memories of the sexual abuse
- not remembering anything (anymore) about the sexual abuse
- not wanting to talk about the sexual abuse:
    - emotional flatness
    - loss of interest
    - daydreaming
    - becoming unattached and estrangement from others (a feeling of being misunderstood by those around you)
    - using substances.

Increased (hyper) vigilance/irritability

- problems with sleeping and staying asleep
- irritability
- concentration problems
- bursts of anger
- risky behaviour
- hyperactive behaviour
- increased jumpy reactions
- physical reactions to triggers that are related to the abuse.

Regressive behaviour

- bed-wetting
- thumb-sucking
- fear of separation.

# Worksheet: Recognising trauma triggers

Many victims of sexual abuse are reminded during their daily lives of the disturbing incident which they have experienced. Often they react to these triggers without being aware of what has caused the reaction.

As parent/caregiver you are the observer of the child or client's behaviour. By constantly asking what, when and where it takes place, it is possible to make a connection between a reminder (trigger) and the trauma. Make a note of this in the observation table below. Pay attention to the presence of people, television programmes, subjects of conversation, names of people, sounds, music, scents and so on.

If it is possible to identify a trauma trigger, appropriate measures can be taken to make sure that the child or client is less often confronted by the trigger.

| Describe the actual behaviour that you see | What happened before this behaviour? | Where does the child/client demonstrate this behaviour? | At which time of day does the child/ client demonstrate this behaviour? |
|---|---|---|---|
| | | | |
| | | | |
| | | | |

# Worksheet: Session preparation

| Session | Are there any changes since the last session? | How are you (both)? | Other issues |
|---|---|---|---|
| 2 | Yes/no | | What do I want to provide for the child/client in the third session? |
| 3 | Yes/no<br><br>If yes, describe the changes... | | |
| 4 | Yes/no<br><br>If yes, describe the changes... | | |

## Worksheet: Session evaluation

| Session | Which important things do I want to remember? | Questions raised during the sessions | Other issues |
|---|---|---|---|
| 1 | | | |
| 2 | | | |
| 3 | | | |
| 4 | | | |

## Form: Name and numbers of helpful people

| Helpful person | Telephone number | Email address | Points of interest |
|---|---|---|---|
| Professional SOS programme | | | |
| Doctor | | | |
| Pharmacy | | | |
| Social worker | | | |
| Police | | | |
| School | | | |
| Victim help | | | |
| Lawyer | | | |
| Law officer | | | |
| | | | |
| | | | |
| | | | |
| | | | |
| | | | |

# Worksheet: SOS evaluation form

Filled in by:

Date and time:

What did you think of the help provided by the SOS programme?

What did you think of the structure of the sessions?

What is the most important thing you will remember about the SOS programme?

Do you have any tips or comments?

# Safety exercises

## Worksheet: Safety agreements

The following safety agreements have been made:

# Worksheet: Safety and reliability[1]

## Instructions for the professional

For a victim of sexual abuse, it is important that clear boundaries and agreements are made. This allows them to regain a grip on daily life. Talk about the safety which will be provided and the reliability of parents and professional caregivers, by using the activities which are a regular part of daily life.

Bathing routines:

- Is the door of the toilet locked when it is used?
- Is the client helped with going to the toilet? If so, in which way?
- Is the door of the shower locked when it is being used?
- Are clients/children washed or showered together?
- Is the client helped with washing and showering? If so, in what way?
- Where and when is the client/child allowed to walk around naked?
- Where and when is a caring adult allowed to walk around naked?

Bed routines:

- Who sleeps with whom in a room? Who sleeps with whom in a bed?
- What are the agreements about people staying the night?
- Where do people get changed and who is present?
- Can bedroom doors be locked?
- Is a goodnight kiss given? If so, where and by whom?

Play fighting and tickling:

- Is it the custom to play fight with or tickle the client/child? If so, how and how often?
- Who is present in that situation?

1 This worksheet is based on Groenbos, Hout and Zon 1996.

- Which body parts are allowed to be touched?
- How do people react if boundaries are crossed?

Internet routines:

- Where are the computers/telephones with an internet connection?
- Is a filter used?
- Are there agreements about internet use? If so, what are these?
- Is internet use of the client checked by others and discussed with them?

Sexual education:

- Are issues such as falling in love, dating, making love, sex, menstruation, ejaculation etc. discussed with the client/child?
- Who talks to whom?
- Which words are used for body parts and sexual activities?

Secrets:

- Is it possible for a client/child to have a secret?
- Is there a difference made between good and bad secrets?
- Are there agreements made about what to do about bad secrets?

# Worksheet: Who needs to know about the abuse and in which way?

| Who? | When? | In which way? | Points of interest |
|---|---|---|---|
| | | | |
| | | | |
| | | | |
| | | | |
| | | | |
| | | | |
| | | | |
| | | | |
| | | | |
| | | | |
| | | | |
| | | | |
| | | | |
| | | | |
| | | | |

# Worries exercise

## Worksheet: Thoughts and feelings

Make cards of the following thoughts and feelings. Put them on a pile and let parents/caregivers take turns reading a card. Ask them to give a reaction to what is written on the card. Give the parent/caregiver the opportunity to pick a different card if they wish to do so.

It is also possible to copy the feelings and thoughts onto an A4 piece of paper. Let those involved make a top ten of the thoughts and feelings which are the most relevant in this situation.

| | |
|---|---|
| I find this an awful subject, one which I would rather not talk about. | I find it difficult to be confronted by the strong emotions of those involved. |
| This can't be true.<br><br>I can't believe it. | I'm scared that previous experiences with sexual abuse will come to the surface again. |
| I doubt whether or not I can cope with this situation. | I'm scared of having to deal with meeting the (suspected) perpetrator. |
| I've got too much on my mind at the moment; I can't deal with this as well. | Why didn't I notice what was going on? I should have prevented this happening. |
| Now you see…I should have listened to my previous suspicions. | It is my fault.<br>I should have noticed. |
| False accusations also happen.<br><br>What if it's not true? | I know the person who has been accused well.<br><br>They wouldn't do such things. |
| … | … |

*Based on Boland* et al.*, 1991.*[1]

1 Boland, G. and Aarnink, G. *et al.* (1991) *Seksueel geweld aan de orde. Werkboek voor het begeleiden van een basis cursus voor hulpverleners*. Utrecht: Medusa.

# Hurt exercise

## Worksheet: My fault or not?[1]

People who are confronted with sexual abuse often feel guilty about the sexual abuse. If this is the case where you are concerned, then can you write here why you think that it is also (partly) your fault?

Can you describe here why you think it is not your fault?

1 Based on Lamers-Winkelman F. (2000) Horizon; 2A. *Een werkboek voor ouders van seksueel misbruikte kinderen*. Amsterdam: SWP.

# Fear exercises

## Worksheet: Scary thoughts

Parents and/or professional caregivers who are confronted with incidents of sexual abuse can be troubled by fearful thoughts. Put a cross on the worksheet next to the thoughts which play a role in your mind, and/or add your own thoughts.

- Will it happen again?

  ______________________________
  ______________________________
  ______________________________
  ______________________________
  ______________________________

- Will my own child become a perpetrator?

  ______________________________
  ______________________________
  ______________________________
  ______________________________
  ______________________________

- Will he/she ever be OK again?

  ______________________________
  ______________________________
  ______________________________
  ______________________________
  ______________________________

- Our child/client has been damaged forever.

  ______________________________
  ______________________________
  ______________________________
  ______________________________
  ______________________________

# Information sheet: How can my child sleep peacefully?

Many children who have experienced bad things do not trust others anymore. They have experienced that it is always possible that bad things will happen everywhere. They are actually always prepared for it to happen again. We call this being alert. If you are always alert, you are not able to relax. If you can't relax then you cannot calm down and it is difficult to sleep.

Another reason why children who have experienced bad things are unable to sleep, is that they have so much time to think about things in the evening and during the night. In the daytime children often look for things to take their mind off it and are busy with other things. In the dark, when they are alone, thoughts, memories and intrusions can occur, in powerful ways.

## Tips for sleeping

1. Check (if possible together with the child) if there are things in the bedroom which remind them of the sexual abuse. You could put the bed in a different place, provide a new quilt cover, or different nightwear.
2. It helps to keep to a fixed sleeping routine: make sure that the child goes to bed at the same time every evening and gets up at the same time in the morning.
3. Develop a relaxing routine for going to sleep: do breathing exercises with the child, listen to peaceful music, put the child in the bath or give them a cup of warm milk or herbal tea.
4. Don't let the child hang around on the sofa or sleep during the daytime – they will sleep badly at night!
5. Let the child use the bed for sleeping only, not for playing on.
6. Make sure that the child gets enough physical exercise every day. However, this should not be just before the child goes to bed! This helps the child to clear their head. Above all, physical movement releases chemicals which make them feel better and helps them to relax!

7. Pay attention to what the child drinks in the evening. Don't let the child eat just before going to bed. Coffee, Coca-Cola and tea keep children awake at night.
8. Make sure that the child's bedroom is clean and tidy; this provides a feeling of calm! The room should not be too warm or too cold – open the window slightly for ventilation. Put on a nightlight if the child likes this.

## Waking up and nightmares

1. If the child wakes up, provide relaxation. Concentrate on breathing, listen to peaceful music or read a (boring) book to them.
2. If the child is troubled by nightmares, name the fear. 'You have been dreaming, you are scared now'. Bring the child into the here and now by saying, 'It is not real, it was just a dream'. If children appear to stay in the dream, ask questions about the here and now, for example what colour the wallpaper or the quilt cover is, or walk to the toilet together.
3. Give the child a safety message, such as, 'All the doors are closed', 'You are safe here', 'Mum and dad are sleeping in the room next to you'.
4. Talk about the dream and bring it to a good end.

# Anger exercise

## Worksheet: I hope I don't meet him anywhere...

Parents/caregivers of children who have experienced sexual abuse from someone nearby often have feelings of anger. The phrase 'I hope I don't meet him anywhere' is often heard. It is good to know in which ways this anger and other feelings can be expressed in a safe way.

My feelings about the incident are:

My thoughts about the incident are:

What can you do to express your anger and other emotions in a safe way?

## Relaxation exercises

### Worksheet: Relaxation and letting go of emotions

What calms you down?

What helps when emotions overwhelm you?

## Exercise: Some relaxation techniques

When the emotions become overwhelming, it is good to know how you can relax. The exercises below can help you with this.

### Counting back from 20 to 0

One way to relax your whole body is by taking long, deep breaths, while slowly counting down from 20 to 0. If possible, close your eyes. Taking long, deep breaths helps to slow down your heartbeat. This relaxes your whole body.

Feel how all the muscles in your body relax further, with every in- and out-breath. Feel the air streaming in through your nose. Feel the breath in your lungs. Feel how your chest and belly fill up with air. Pay attention to how your belly expands on the in-breath. Follow the out-breath, feel your belly and chest emptying of air. Feel how the out-breath streams out through your nose.

Do 20 of these in- and out-breaths. Then you will feel well and relaxed.

### Breathe in and relaxxxxx

Sit down with a straight back. Breathe in through your nose (for about three counts 1...2...3...) and count slowly while breathing out (4...5...6...7...8...9...10...).

Do this three times.

Also try thinking (breathe IN...) and Relaxxxxxx (on the out-breath).

### Send your thoughts to your body

- Sit upright on your chair, feet on the ground.
- Breathe calmly.
- Close your eyes and concentrate.
- Send your thoughts to:
  - your feet (and feel how they are positioned on the ground)
  - your ankles
  - your knees
  - your thighs
  - your belly (feel your breath)

- your back from the bottom to the top
- your shoulder blades
- the tops of your arms
- the bottom of your arms
- your wrists
- your fingers
- slowly back to your shoulders
- your neck
- your head
- your ears
- your cheeks
- your eyes.

## Muscle tension and relaxation

Do the same as in exercise 'Send your thoughts to your body', but first tense the muscle you are thinking of and then let go.

So at each part of your body, tense and relax.

## Imagination exercises

Breathe in and out. Imagine that you are sitting in a place where you feel pleasant. This works best with eyes closed.

- What does it look like?
- Where are you?
- Who are you with?
- What are you doing?
- How are you feeling?

Go to this place in your imagination every time you feel bad.

## Breathing exercises

- Sit up straight: upright, feet on the ground.
- Breathe in very slowly and deeply through your nose (three seconds), expanding your belly.
- Breathe out calmly through your mouth (three seconds).

## Worksheet: Support from people around you

Please fill in the people who can support you and fill in the way in which they can do this.

| People around me | These people can support me in this way |
|---|---|
| | |
| | |
| | |
| | |
| | |
| | |

## Worksheet: And now me!

What would you like to do for yourself?

In which way will you succeed in doing this?

# ABOUT THE AUTHORS

**Aafke Scharloo MSc** is a clinical psychologist and remedial educationalist. She began in the late 1980s as a pioneer in the approach to sexual abuse in people with an intellectual disability and has been involved in this subject ever since. Aafke is one of the designers of the method of minimum fact interviews in suspicions of sexual abuse in the Netherlands and works throughout the country as an expert for healthcare professionals, parents and clients themselves. She also works with the police and justice system on issues concerning this subject. Alongside substantive clinical work, Aafke also works as an educator, trainer, superviser and adviser. Aafke gives national and international lectures and publishes articles in journals and books. She is independently established and specialises in issues concerning people with an intellectual disability, sexual abuse, maltreatment and trauma.

**Simone Ebbers-Mennink MSc** is a healthcare psychologist, remedial educationalist and sexologist. Simone has been working for years in secondary and higher vocational education. In 2002, she wrote a study book on sexuality and sexual abuse for care-providing professions. Since 2003, she has been working as a professional within remedial education treatment centre Vitree with children and teenagers with a mild intellectual disability and psychiatric issues. Simone specialises in diagnostics and therapy regarding sexual abuse and trauma and is an expert on sexuality. In addition, she works in her own practice for primary psychological care, which focuses on children and teenagers with issues concerning sexuality, sexual abuse and trauma.

**Martine Spijker-van Vuren MSc** is a healthcare psychologist and EMDR therapist and practitioner. Martine has been working since 1998 in the care for people with a mild intellectual disability.

She is one of the founders of the expertise centre of the remedial education centre Ambiq in Hengelo. This expertise centre conducts diagnostics and treatment for children and young adults with a mild intellectual disability and trauma-related symptoms and sexual behaviour issues. In addition, she works in her own practice for primary psychological care in which, alongside treating general psychological complaints, she also specialises in trauma, sexuality and sexual abuse in children, teenagers and (young) adults.

# NOTES

## Foreword

1. Došen, A., Gennep, A. van, Zwanniken, G. (1990) 'Treatment of mental illness and behavioural disorder in the mentally retarded.' Proceedings of the International Congress, 3–4 May, Amsterdam, Logon, Leiden.
2. Bowlby, J. (1979) 'On knowing what you are not supposed to know and feeling what you are not supposed to feel.' *The Canadian Journal of Psychiatry 24,* 403–408.
3. Ferenczi, S. (1928) *Final Contributions to the Problems and Methods of Psychoanalysis.* Michael Balint (ed.) (1955) *The Elasticity of Psychoanalytical Techniques.* London. Hogarth Press.
4. Sinason, V. (1986) 'Secondary mental handicap and its relationship to trauma.' *Psychoanalytic psychotherapy* 2 (2), 131–154.
5. Sinason, V. (2012) *Mental Handicap and the Human Condition: A Psychoanalytic Approach to Intellectual Disability,* revised 2nd edition. UK: Free Association Books.

## Chapter 1

1. Scharloo, A. and Bors, J. (2012) *Onbestaanbaar waar.* Oplo: De Seizoenen.
2. Berlie, E. de, Ivens, C., Lesseliers L., Hove, G. van (red.) (2000) *Seksueelmisbruik en mensen met een verstandelijke handicap.* Leusden: Acco.
3. Pynoos, R. S. (1996) *Caring for Children Who Have Experienced Trauma.* Los Angeles: National Child Traumatic Stress Network.
4. Briere, J. and Scott, C. (2006) *Principles of Trauma Therapy: A Guide to Symptoms, Evaluation and Treatment.* Thousand Oaks, CA: Sage Publications.
5. Berlo, W. van, *et al.* (2011) *Beperkt weerbaar – een onderzoek naar seksueel geweld bij mensen een lichamelijke, zintuiglijke of verstandelijke beperking.* Utrecht: Rutgers WPF/ Movisie.
6. Cottis, C. (2009) 'Love Hurts: The Emotional Impact of Intellectual Disability and Sexual Abuse on a Family.' In C. Cottis (ed.) *Intellectual Disability, Trauma and Psychotherapy.* London: Routledge.
7. Pynoos 1996.
8. Brugsteden, R. van, Heestermans, M., Swennen, M. (2011) *Seksualiteit en seksueel misbruik en Sturen op aanpak van seksueel misbruik.* Utrecht: VGN en keenisplein gehandicaptenzorg.
9. van Kuban, C. and Steele, W. (2008) In *One-minute Interventions for Traumatized Children and Adolescents.* Detroit: TLC Institute.

## Chapter 2

1. Gill, C. J. (2010) 'No, we don't think our doctors are out to get us: Responding to the straw man distortions of disability rights arguments against assisted suicide.' *Disability and Health Journal,* 3, 31–38.

2. McCarthy, M. and Thompson, D. (1996) 'Sexual abuse by design.' *Disability & Society,* 11 (2), 205–218. London: Routledge.
3. McCarthy M. and Thompson D. (eds) (2010) *Sexuality and Learning Disabilities.* Brighton: Pavilion Publishing.
4. Nicolai, N. J. (1997) 'Over splitsen, splijten en dissociëren.' *Tijdschrift voor Psychotherapie* 23, 46–58.
5. Brugsteden, R. van, Heestermans, M. and Swennen, M. (2011) *Seksualiteit en seksueel misbruik en Sturen op aanpak van seksueel misbruik.* Utrecht: VGN en kennisplein gehandicaptenzorg.
6. Turey-Wijne, I. (2013) *How to Break the Bad News to People with Intellectual Disabilities – A Guide for Carers and Professionals.* London: Jessica Kingsley Publishers.
7. Brugsteden, R. *et al.* 2011.
8. WGBO artikel 7:465 lid 2.
9. Werkgroep Ministerie van Justitie (2007) *Handreiking voor de beoordeling van wilsonbekwaamheid.* 's Gravenhage: Ministerie van Justitie.
10. Appelbaum, P. S. and Grisso, T. (1988) 'Assessing patients' capacities to consent to treatment.' *New England Journal of Medicine,* 319, 1635–1638.
11. Rozee, P. and Koss, M. (2001) 'Rape: a century of resistance.' *Psychology of Woman Quarterly,* 25, 295–311.
12. Garcia-Moreno, C., Jansen, H., Ellsberg, M., Heise, L. and Watts, C. (2005) *WHO Multi-Country Study on Women's Health and Domestic Violence Against Women.* Geneva: WHO Library Catalogen.
13. Johnson, H., Ollus, N. and Nevala, S. (2008) *Violence Against Women: An International Perspective.* New York: Springer.
14. Lalor, K. and McElvaney, R. (2010) 'Child sexual abuse, links to later sexual exploitation/ high risk sexual behaviour and prevention/treatment programs.' *Trauma, Violence & Abuse,* 11 (4), 159–177.
15. Bakker, F., Graaf, H. de, Haas, S. de, Kedde, H., Kruijer, H. and Wijsen, C. (2009) *Seksuele gezondheid in Nederland.* Utrecht: Rutgers Nisso groep.
16. Portegijs, W., Hermans, B. and Lalba, V. (2006) *Emancipatiemonitor 2006. Veranderingen in de leefsituatie en levensloop.* Den Haag: SCP.
17. Baladarian, N. (1991) 'Sexual abuse of people with developmental disabilities.' *Journal of Sexuality and Disability,* 9 (4), 323–335.
18. Sobsey, D. and Doe, T. (1991) 'Patterns of sexual abuse and assault.' *Sexuality and Disability,* 9 (3), 243–259.
19. Gorman-Smith, D. and Matson, J. L. (1992) 'Sexual Abuse and Persons with Developmental Disabilities.' In W. T. O'Donohue and A. Geer (eds) *The Sexual Abuse of Children: Theory, Research, and Therapy 12.* Hillsdale, NJ: Lawrence-Erlbaum Association.
20. Westat Inc. (1991/1993) *A Report on the Maltreatment of Children with Disabilities.* Washington DC: US Department of Health and Human Services.
21. Gordon, B. N. and Schroeder, C. S. (1995) *Sexuality: A Developmental Approach to Problems.* New York: Plenum Publishing Corp.
22. Hingsberger, D. and Melberg Schwier, K. (2000) *Sexuality, Your Sons and Daughters with Intellectual Disabilities.* London: Jessica Kingsley Publishers.
23. Berlo, W. van *et al.* (2011*) Beperkt weerbaar – een onderzoek naar seksueel geweld bij mensen met een lichamelijke, zintuiglijke of verstandelijke beperking.* Utrecht: Rutgers WPF/Movisie.
24. Duke, J. E. A. (2006) *Summary of Literature on Sexual Violence Against People with Development Disabilities.* Oregon: Public Health Division.
25. Belie, E. de, Ivens, C., Lesseliers, J. and Hove, G. van (red.) (2000) *Seksueel misbruik en mensen met een verstan-delijke handicap.* Leusden: Acco.
26. Commissie Samson (2012) *Omringd door zorg, toch niet veilig. Seksueel misbruik van door de overheid uit huis geplaatste kinderen, 1945-heden.* Amsterdam: Boom.
27. Commissie Samson 2012.
28. Spanjaard, H., Haspels, M. and Roos, I. (2000) 'Grenzen stellen en respecteren: onderzoek naar de e ecten van programmaontwikkeling omtrent seksualiteit.' *Nederlands tijdschrift voor Zwakzinnigenzorg, 26* (4), 211–228.
29. Crosse, S. B., Kaye, E. and Ratnofsky, A. C. (1993) *A report on the maltreatment of children with disabilities.* Washington DC: National Center on Child Abuse and Neglect, DHHS.

30. Sullivan, P. M. and Knutson, J. F. (1998) 'The association between maltreatment and disabilities in a hospital-based epidemiologic study.' *Child Abuse Neglect,* 22, 271.
31. Classen, C. C., Palesh, O. G. and Aggerwal, R. (2005) 'Sexual revictimization: A review of the emperical literature.' *Trauma, Violence and Abuse,* 6 (2), 103–129.
32. Baladarian 1991.
33. Berlo *et al.* 2011.
34. Turk, V. and Brown, H. (1993) 'The sexual abuse of adults with learning disabilities: Results of a two-year incidence survey.' *Mental Handicap Research,* 6, 193–216.
35. Sobsey, D. (1994) *Violence and Abuse in the Lives of People with Disabilities – The End of the Silent Acceptance.* Baltimore: Pal H. Brookes Publishing Company.
36. Finkelhor, D. and Asdigian, N. L. (1996) 'Risk factors for youth victimization: Beyond a lifestyles/routine activities theory approach.' *Violence & victims,* 11, 3–20.
37. Berlo, W. van (1995) *Seksueel misbruik bij mensen met een verstandelijke handicap.* Delft: Eburon.
38. Berlo *et al.* 2011.
39. Sobsey and Doe 1991.
40. Commissie Samson 2012.
41. Berlo *et al.* 2011.
42. Sobsey 1994.
43. Scharloo, A. (2009) *Kwetsbaar: Kinderen met een beperking, een vergeten groep met onzichtbare slachto ers.* Uitgeest: Tijdschrift kindermishandeling.
44. Berlo 1995.
45. TransAct (2005) Utrecht.
46. Berlo, W. van and Put, C. van der, genoemd in Kersten (2003) Kersten, M., *Seksualiteit van mensen met een handicap. Een analyse van bestaande kennis en aanwijzingen voor praktijk en verdere kennisverwerving.* Utrecht: LKNG.
47. Finkelhor, D. (1986) *A Sourcebook on Child Sexual Abuse.* Beverly Hills, CA: Sage Publications.
48. Brown, H., Hunt, N. and Stein, J. (1994) 'Alarming but very necessary: Working with staff groups around the sexual abuse of adults with learning disabilities.' *Mental Handicap,* 20, 44–55.
49. Douma, J., Bergh, P. and Hoekman, J. van den (1998) *Verstandelijk gehandicapten en seksueel misbruik.* Rotterdam: Lemniscaat.
50. Lewis, L., Kelly, K. and Allen, J. (2004) *Restoring Hope And Trust: An Illustrated Guide To Mastering Trauma.* Brooklandville, MD: Sidran Institute Press.
51. Cense, M. (1997) *Rode kaart of carte blanche; risicofactoren voor seksuele intimidatie en seksueel misbruik in de sport.* Arnhem: NOC*NSF.
52. Finkelhor, D. (1984) *Child Sexual Abuse: New Theory and Research.* New York: The Free Press.
53. Mastenbroek, S. (1995) *De illusie van veiligheid.* Utrecht: Jan van Arkel.
54. Commissie Samson 2012.
55. Belie *et al.* 2000.
56. Scharloo, A. (2005) *Seksueel misbruik: de gevolgen voor ouders en verwanten.* Utrecht: VOGG Raakpunt.
57. Scharloo 2005.
58. National Child Traumatic Stress Network (2010) *Caring for Children who have Experienced Trauma, Participant Handbook.* Los Angeles: NCTSN.
59. Berlo *et al.* 2011.
60. Turk and Brown 1993.
61. Sobsey 1994.
62. Finkelhor and Asdigian 1996.
63. National Child Traumatic Stress Network 2010.
64. Slachtofferhulp (2003) *Kinderen helpen na een schokkende gebeurtenis; praktische gids na een misdrijf of plots overlijden.* Houten: Lannoo.
65. Belie *et al.* 2000.
66. National Child Traumatic Stress Network (2009) *Caring for Kids: What Parents Need to Know about Sexual Abuse.* Los Angeles: NCTSN.

67. Scharloo, A. (2012) *Seksuele opvoeding bij kinderen met seksueel misbruik ervaringen. Congres opvoeden van getraumatiseerde kinderen.* Houten: Bohn Sta eu van Loghum.
68. Johnson, T. C. (1998) *Sexuality Curriculum for Abused Children and Young Adolescents and their Parents.* Pasadena, CA: Cavanagh Johnson.


## Chapter 3


1. www.IGZ.nl.
2. Deze wijziging in de Kwaliteitswet zorginstellingen is gedaan in juni 2005.
3. Inspectie voor de Gezondheidszorg (2004) Het mag niet, het mag nooit, seksuele intimidatie door hulpverleners in de gezondheidszorg. Den Haag: Inspectie voor de Gezondheidszorg.
4. Jeugdzorgwet, artikel 21.
5. Brugsteden, R. van, Heestermans, M. and Swennen, M. (2011) *Seksualiteit en seksueel misbruik en Sturen opaanpak van seksueel misbruik.* Utrecht: VGN en kennisplein gehandicaptenzorg.
6. WGBO, artikel 450, lid 2 BW.
7. WGBO, artikel 450, lid 2 BW.
8. WGBO, artikel 447 BW.
9. WGBO, artikel 450, lid 2 BW.
10. WGBO, artikel 465, lid 4 BW.
11. WGBO artikel 466, lid 1 BW.
12. WGBO, artikel 456 BW.
13. WGBO, artikel 457 BW.
14. WGBO, artikel 7:448 lid 1 BW.
15. WGBO, artikel 1:377b BW.
16. WGBO, artikel 7:457 lid 1 BW, artikel 88 Wet BIG, artikel 9 lid 4 WBP.
17. Wet op de jeugdzorg, artikel 53 lid 3.
18. Wetboek van strafrecht, artikel 40.
19. Wetboek van Strafvordering, artikel 218.
20. VGN notitie: Medisch beroepsgeheim en verschoningsrecht in de gehandicaptenzorg.
21. www.huiselijkgeweldenberoepsgeheim.nl, de digitale wegwijzer huiselijk geweld, kindermishandelingen beroepsgeheim: 'Horen, zien en zwijgplicht' van het ministerie van justitie.
22. Brugsteden, Heestermans and Swennen 2011.
23. Openbaar Ministerie (2011) Aanwijzing opsporing en vervolging inzake seksueel misbruik.
24. Openbaar Ministerie (2011) Aanwijzing opsporing en vervolging inzake seksueel misbruik.
25. www.LANZS.nl.
26. Lammers, M. and Goes, A. (2006) *Van incident tot fundament; vormgeving en implementatie van beleid rondbejegening, seksualiteit en seksueel misbruik.* Utrecht: MOVISIE/Transact.
27. www.polikindermishandeling.nl.
28. Kinderen jeugdtraumacentrum (2004) *Folder: Medisch onderzoek bij een vermoeden van seksueel misbruik.* Haarlem: Kinder-en jeugdtraumacentrum.


## Chapter 4


1. American Psychiatric Association (2013) *Diagnostic and Statistical Manual of Mental Disorders-fifth edition.*
2. Aarts, P. G. H. and Visser, W. D. (2007) *Trauma, diagnostiek en behandeling.* Houten: Bohn Stafleu van Loghum.
3. Coppens, L. and Kregten, C. van (2012) *Zorgen voor getraumatiseerde kinderen: een training voor opvoeders. Handboek voor trainers.* Houten: Bohn Stafleu van Loghum.
4. Terr, L. C. (1991) 'Childhood traumas: an outline and overview.' *American Journal of Psychiatry,* 148, 10–20.

5. Coppens, L. and Kregten, C. van (2012) *Zorgen voor getraumatiseerde kinderen: een training voor opvoeders. Handboek voor trainers.* Houten: Bohn Stafleu van Loghum.
6. Figley, P. H. D. and Charles R. (1995) *Compassion Fatigue: Coping with Secondary Stress Disorder in those who Treat the Traumatized.* New York and London: Brunner-Routledge.
7. Figley, P. H. D. and Charles R. (1995) *Compassion Fatigue: Coping with Secondary Stress Disorder in those who Treat the Traumatized.* New York and London: Brunner-Routledge.
8. Teicher, M. H. (2002) *Scars That Won't Heal: The Neurobiology of Child Abuse.* New York: Scientific American Inc.
9. Perry. B. D. (2000) *The neuroarcheology of childhood maltreatment: the neurodevelopmental costs of adverse childhood events.* Available at www.childtrauma.org.
10. Perry, B. and Szalavitz, M. (2007) *De jongen die opgroeide als een hond.* Schiedam: Scriptum psychologie.
11. Eland, J., Roos, C. de and Kleber, R. (2000) *Kind en trauma; een opvangprogramma.* Lisse: Swets & Zeitlinger.
12. Coppens and Kregten 2012.
13. Bicanic, I. (2002) 'Geweld in de hersenen; de neurobiologische gevolgen van kindermishandeling.' *Tijdschrift Kinder en jeugdpsychiatrie* 29 (3), 33–45.
14. Struik, A. (2010) *Slapende honden? Wakker maken! Een stabilisatiemethode voor chronisch getraumatiseerde kinderen.* Amsterdam: Pearson.
15. Cohen, J. A., Mannarino, A.P. and Deblinger, E. (2008) *Behandeling van trauma bij kinderen en adolescenten.* Houten: Bohn Stafleu van Loghum.
16. Coppens and Kregten 2012.
17. Putnam, F. W. (1997) *Dissociation in Children and Adolescents: A Developmental Perspective.* New York: The Guilford Press.
18. Coppens and Kregten 2012.
19. Weringh, E. van (2003) Het begrijpen van effecten van mishandeling op de vroege ontwikkeling van hersenen (vertaling van: In *Focus © Administration for Children and Families* (2001); US Department of Health and Human Services). Rotterdam: Stichting Empty Memories.
20. Perry, B. D. (2002) 'Childhood experience and the expression of genetic potential: what childhood neglect tells us about nurture and nature.' *Brain and mind,* 3, 79–100.
21. Perry and Szalavitz 2007.
22. Ito, Y., Teicher, M. H., Glod, C. A. *et al.* (1998) 'Preliminary evidence for aberrant cortical development. Abused children; a quantitive EEG-study.' *Journal of Neuropsychiatry and Clinical Neurosciences,* 10, 298–307.
23. Verdouw 2009.
24. Emmerik, A. van and Berretty, E. (2007) *Leven met een trauma.* Houten: Bohn Stafleu van Loghum.
25. Coppens and Kregten 2012.
26. Eland, J., Roos, C. de and Kleber, R. (2000) *Kind en trauma; een opvangprogramma.* Lisse: Swets & Zeitlinger.
27. Hart, O. van der (1991) *Trauma: dissociatie en hypnose.* Lisse: Swets & Zeitlinger.
28. Struik, A. 2010.
29. Schäfer, I., Barkmann, C., Riedesser, P. and Schulte-Markwort, M. (2004) 'Peritraumatic dissociation predicts post-traumatic stress in children and adolescents following road traffic accidents.' *Journal of Trauma & Dissociation,* 5 (4), 79–91.
30. Putnam, F. W. (1993) *An Update on the Child Dissociative Checklist.* Lisse: Swetz & Zeitlinger.
31. Deering, C. G., Glover, S.G., Ready, D., Eddleman, H. C., Alarcon, R. D. (1996) 'Unique patterns of comorbidity in posttraumatic stress disorder from different sources of trauma.' *Comprehensive Psychiatry,* 37 (5), 336–346.
32. Aarts, P. G. H. and Visser, W. D. (2007) *Trauma, diagnostiek en behandeling.* Houten: Bohn Stafleu van Loghum.
33. Emmerik and Berretty 2007.
34. Aarts and Visser 2007.

35. Oldham, J. M., Riba, M.B. and Tasman, A. (1993) 'Pynoos traumatic stress and developmental psychopathology in children and adolescents.' *EDS, American Psychiatric Press Review of Psychiatry,* 12, 205–237.
36. Putnam, F. W. (1997) *Dissociation in Children and Adolescents: A Developmental Perspective.* New York: The Guildford Press.
37. Alisic, E. (2012) *Kinderen ondersteunen na trauma.* Amsterdam: Boom.
38. Cohen, J. A. and Mannarino, A. P. (1998) 'Factors that mediate treatment outcome of sexually abused preschool children: six- and 12-month follow-up.' *Journal of the American Academy of Child and Adolescent Psychiatry,* 37, 44–51.
39. Perrin, S., Smith, P. and Yule, W. (2000) 'The assessment and treatment of Post-traumatic Stress Disorder in children and adolescents.' *Journal of Child Psychology and Psychiatry, and allied disciplines,* 41, 277–289.
40. Joshi, P. T. and O'Donnell, D. A. (2003) 'Consequences of child exposure to war and terrorism.' *Clinical Child and Family Psychology Review,* 6, 275–292.
41. Perrin, Smith and Yule 2000.
42. Terr, L. C. (1991) 'Childhood traumas – an outline and overview.' *American Journal of Psychiatry,* 148, 10–20.
43. Adler Nevo, G. and Manassis, K. (2005) 'Psychosocial treatment of pediatric posttraumatic stress disorder: the neglected field of single-incident trauma.' *Depression and Anxiety,* 22, 177–189.
44. Cohen J. A., Mannarino, A. P. and Deblinger, E. (2008) *Behandeling van trauma bij kinderen en adolescenten.* Houten: Bohn Stafleu van Loghum.
45. Lindauer, R. and Boer, F. (2012) *Trauma bij kinderen, kinderpsychologie in praktijk.* Houten: Lannoo Campus.
46. Lindauer and Boer 2012.
47. Slachtofferhulp (2003) *Kinderen helpen na een schokkende gebeurtenis; praktische gids na een misdrijf of plots overlijden.* Houten: Lannoo.
48. Mittendorf, C. and Muller, E. (2010) *Ik ben er kapot van. Over psychotrauma en de verwerking van schokkende gebeurtenissen.* Amsterdam: Boom.
49. Berlo, W. van, *et al.* (2011) *Beperkt weerbaar – een onderzoek naar seksueel geweld bij mensen met een lichamelijke, zintuiglijke of verstandelijke beperking.* Utrecht: Rutgers WPF/ Movisie.
50. Sequera, H. and Hollins, S. (2003) 'Clinical effects of sexual abuse on people with learning disabilities.' *British Journal of Psychiatry,* 182, 13–19.
51. Sequera and Hollins 2003.
52. Fletcher R. *et al.* (2007) *DM-ID: Diagnostic, Manual-Intellectual Disability.* New York: NADD.
53. Fletcher *et al.* 2007.
54. Dösen, A. (2005) *Psychische stoornissen, gedragsproblemen verstandelijke handicap.* Assen: Van Gorcum.
55. Macklin, M. L., Litz, B. T. and Mc Nally, R. J. (2007) 'Lower precombat intelligence is a risk factor for post traumatic stress.' *Journal of Consulting and Clinical Psychology,* 20, 657–666.
56. Dösen 2005.
57. Boon, S., Steel, K. and Hart, O. van der (2012) *Omgaan met traumagerelateerde dissociatie.* Amsterdam: Pearson.
58. Sinason, V. (2010) *Mental Handicap and the Human Condition.* London: FA Books.
59. Sinason 2010.
60. McCarthey, M. (1999) *Sexuality and Women with Learning Disabilities.* Gateshead: Athenaeum Press.
61. IJzendoorn, M. H. van, *et al.* (2010) *Gehechtheid en trauma, diagnostiek en behandeling voor de professional.* Amsterdam: Hogrefe Uitgevers.
62. Sinason 2010.
63. De Belie, E. and Morisse, F. (red.) (2006) *Gehechtheid en gehechtheidsproblemen bij personen met een verstandelijke beperking.* Apeldoorn: Garant.
64. Greenwald, R. (2005) *Child Trauma Handbook. A Guide for Helping Trauma-Exposed Children and Adolescents.* New York: Routledge.

65. Boon, Steel and Hart 2012.
66. McCarthey 1999.
67. Struik 2010.
68. Hart, O. van der, Nijenhuis, E. and Steele, K. (2006) *Het belaagde zelf.* Amsterdam: Boom.
69. Scharloo, A. (2012) *Trauma Treatment with People with Developmental Disabilities After Abuse.* Long Beach: ISSTD.
70. Sinason (2010) ISSTD Conference.
71. Mevisssen, L., Lievegoed, R. and Jongh, A. de (2010) 'EMDR treatment in people with mild ID and PTSD: 4 cases.' *The Psychiatric Quarterly,* 82 (1), 43–57.
72. Scharloo 2012.
73. Boon, S. and Draaijer, N. (1998) *Screening en diagnostiek van dissociatieve stoornissen.* Lisse: Swets & Zeitlinger.

## Chapter 5

1. Detavernier, B. (2011) 'De grens voorbij.' In *Hulpverlening bij kindermishandeling.* Antwerpen: Garant.
2. National Child Traumatic Stress Network (2006) *Psychological First Aid, Field Operations Guide.* Los Angeles: NCTSN.
3. Ogden, P. (2012) *Trauma and the Body.* Long Beach: ISSTD.
4. Perry, B. (2007) *De jongen die opgroeide als een hond (en andere verhalen uit de kinderpsychiatrische praktijk).* New York: Basic books.
5. Siegel, D. (2010) *Mindsight, De psychologie van het nieuwe bewustzijn.* Houten: Unieboek, het Spectrum.
6. Dorrepaal, E., Thomaes, K. and Draaier, N. (2009) *Vroeger en verder.* Amsterdam: Pearson.
7. National Child Traumatic Stress Network 2006.
8. Briere, J. and Scott, C. (2006) *Principles of Trauma Therapy; A Guide to Symptoms, Evaluation and Treatment.* Thousand Oaks, CA: Sage Publications.
9. Dolan, Y. M. and Craemer, L. de (2005) *Omgaan met seksueel misbruik: oplossingsgerichte therapie en Ericksonlaanse hypnose voor volwassenen.* Amsterdam: Harcourt.
10. Pynoos, R. S. (1996) *Caring for Children who have Experienced Trauma.* Los Angeles: National Child Traumatic Stress Network.
11. van Kuban, C., and Steele, W. (2008) In *One minute Interventions for Traumatized Children and Adolescents.* Detroit: TLC-institute.

## Chapter 6

1. Sinason, V. (2010) *Mental Handicap and the Human Condition.* London: FA Books.
2. Berlo, W. van, *et al.* (2011) *Beperkt weerbaareen onderzoek naar seksueel geweld bij mensen met een lichamelijke, zintuiglijke of verstandelijke beperking.* Utrecht: Rutgers WPF/Movisie.
3. Sinason 2010.
4. Vrij naar: Delfos, M. (1994) 'De ontwikkeling van intimiteit, een ontwikkelingspsychologisch model, gekoppeld aan een model van de gevolgen van seksueel misbruik.' *Tijdschrift voor Seksuologie,* 18 (4), 282–292.

## Chapter 7

1. Zon, A. van (2010) 'Ik wil ook' –; Leren in kinderdagcentra. Antwerpen: Garant.
2. Hewitt, S. K. (2007) 'Brief screening for sexual abuse in very young children.' San Diego: conference.
3. Rothschild, B. (2000) *The Body Remembers: the Psychophysiology of Trauma and Trauma Treatment.* New York: Norton7Company.

4. Corbett, A. (2009) 'Words as Second Language – The Psychotherapeutic Challenge of Severe Intellectual Disability.' In T. Cottis (ed.) *Intellectual Disability, Trauma and Psychotherapy.* London: Routledge.
5. Sherborne developmental movement (www.sherbornovementuk.org). Marsden, E. and Egerton, J. (2007) *Moving with Research.* Sunfield Publications.

## Chapter 8

1. In this chapter we have chosen to refer to victims as children, in order to benefit the readability of the text. In real life, it can be that the child has already reached an adult age. The SOS programme can be used for victims of all ages.
2. Cottis, C. (2009) 'Love Hurts: The Emotional Impact of Intellectual Disability and Sexual Abuse on a Family.' In C. Cottis (ed.) *Intellectual Disability, Trauma and Psychotherapy.* London: Routledge.
3. Scharloo, A. (2005) *Seksueel misbruik: de gevolgen voor ouders en verwanten.* Utrecht: VOGG Raakpunt.
4. Duke, J. (2004) *Factsheet on children with developmental disabilities.* Los Angeles: National Child Traumatic Stress Network.
5. Scharloo 2005.
6. Eland, J., Roos, C. de and Kleber, R. (2000) *Kind en trauma; een opvangprogramma.* Lisse: Swets & Zeitlinger.
7. National Child Traumatic Stress Network (2009) *Caring for Kids; What Parents Need to Know About Sexual Abuse.* Los Angeles: NCTSN.
8. National Child Traumatic Stress Network 2009.
9. Wasserman, B. (2005) *Feeling Good Again: A Guide for Parents and Therapists of Sexually Abused Children.* Brandon: The safer society press.
10. Slachtofferhulp (2003) *Kinderen helpen na een schokkende gebeurtenis; praktische gids na een misdrijf of plots overlijden.* Houten: Lannoo.
11. Federatie pleegzorg (1996) *Omgaan met een seksueel misbruikt kind: een cursus voor pleegouders.* Amsterdam: Federatie pleegzorg, Hogeschool van Amsterdam, Stichting therapeutische gezinsverpleging.
12. Wasserman 2005.
13. Brohl, K. (2004) *When Your Child Has Been Molested.* San Francisco: Jossey-Bass.
14. Brohl 2004.
15. Brohl 2004.
16. Greenwald, R. (2005) *Child Trauma Handbook. A Guide for helping Trauma-Exposed Children and Adolescents.* New York: Routledge.
17. Schwab, Z. F. (2002) *Beide benen op de grond; keuzes maken na een zedendelict.* Capelle aan den IJssel: Uitgeverij Schwab.

## Chapter 9

1. Green, B. L. *et al.* (1991) 'Children and disaster: age, gender and parental effects on PTSD symptoms.' *Journal of the American Academy of Child and Adolescent Psychiatry,* 30, 945–951.
2. Douma, J., Bergh, P. and Hoekman, J. van den (1998) *Verstandelijk gehandicapten en seksueel misbruik.* Rotterdam: Lemniscaat.
3. Bosch, E. and Suykerbuyk, E. (2005) *Begeleiding van seksueel misbruikte mensen met een verstandelijke handicap.* Amsterdam: Nelissen.
4. Eeland, K. and Woelinga, H. (1991) *Praktische richtlijnen voor de hulpverlening bij seksueel misbruik van kinderen. Amsterdam: VU.*
5. Coppens, L. and Kregten, C. van (2012) *Zorgen voor getraumatiseerde kinderen: een training voor opvoeders. Handboek voor trainers.* Houten: Bohn Stafleu van Loghum.

6. Briere, J. and Scott, C. (2006) *Principles of Trauma Therapy: A Guide to Symptoms, Evaluation and Treatment.* Thousand Oaks, CA: Sage Publications.
7. Mittendorf, C. and Mulller, E. (2010) *Ik ben er kapot van.* Amsterdam: Boom.
8. Eland, J., Roos, C. de and Kleber, R. (2000) *Kind en trauma; een opvangprogramma.* Lisse: Swets & Zeitlinger.
9. Douma, Bergh and Hoekman 1998.
10. Bosch and Suykerbuyk 2005.
11. Pruijssers, A. (2008) *Ik wordtsoms boos, maar dan ben ik bang.* Gouda: CCE.
12. Garmezy, N. (1985) cited in Rutter (1987) 'Psychological resiliende and protective mechanisms.' *American Journal of Orthopsychiatry,* 57, 316–331.
13. Kroef, M. (okt.1995) Iedereen staat op z'n benen te trillen. Capelle a/d IJssel: Klik, 12–14.
14. Brugsteden, R. van, Heestermans, M. and Swennen, M. (2011) *Seksualiteit en seksueel misbruik en Sturen opaanpak van seksueel misbruik.* Utrecht: VGN en kennisplein gehandicaptenzorg.
15. Korven, A. van (1999) Het verwoestende proces bij splitting. Is er iets aan te doen? Oostmalle: Workshop tijdens de inservicedagen van het Opleidings Centrum Autisme, Tripode casemanagement cursussen en advies.
16. Delft, F. van (2004) *Overdracht en tegenoverdracht – een therapeutisch fenomeen vertaald naar alledaagse psychosociale begeleiding.* Soest: Nelissen.
17. Coppens and Kregten 2012.